Retinal and Optic Nerve Stem Cell Surgery

Jeffrey N. Weiss

Retinal and Optic Nerve Stem Cell Surgery

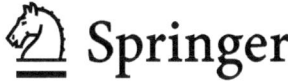 Springer

Jeffrey N. Weiss
Parkland, FL
USA

ISBN 978-3-030-60852-1   ISBN 978-3-030-60850-7   (eBook)
https://doi.org/10.1007/978-3-030-60850-7

This Springer imprint is published by the registered company Springer Nature Switzerland AG
The registered company address is: Gewerbestrasse 11, 6330 Cham, Switzerland

To the patients that have allowed me the privilege to serve.

Preface

Over the last 30 years, we have heard about stem cells and the possibility that they may treat presently untreatable and blinding retinal and optic nerve diseases.

There have been animal studies, companies perform small studies and then disappear, but nothing concrete has materialized. The FDA has repeatedly changed their regulations precluding the stability businesses require for investing. Companies must develop a proprietary product or process that allows them to recoup their investment and earn a profit.

What if a proprietary product is not necessary? What if the solution is simple? How could that be brought to the market? There is much misinformation in our journals that speak about this work but know nothing about it.

I began working in the stem cell field in 2009. I performed retinal stem cell surgery on two American patients in Germany in 2010, seven American patients in Austria in 2011, and, finally, in the U.S.A in 2012. I have now performed the surgery on more than 500 patients in the U.S.

In this book, I provide the basis and details, the protocols, informed consents, and other information that would be helpful to a physician or researcher interested in this work.

I value your constructive opinions and comments.

Parkland, FL, USA   Jeffrey N. Weiss

Contents

Chapter 1
Stem Cells, PRP, Definitions, FDA

Stem cells are undifferentiated cells capable of self-renewal (reproduction) and are capable of producing specific types of cells, a process known as differentiation.

Embryonic stem cells, extracted from blastocysts, may be stimulated to differentiate into specific cell types. In the developing embryo, these cells differentiate into ectoderm, endoderm, and mesoderm. Embryonic cells can differentiate into any type of cell, but this can be disadvantageous, as they can form tumors. Much of the early stem cell research was performed using this type of cell. Because of the source of their derivation, there has been much religious and moral controversy.

Induced pluripotent stem cells are differentiated, or older cells, that can be stimulated to return to an undifferentiated state. This would create an inexhaustible supply of cells but mutations in the cell line may be a problem.

Adult stem cells are found in cord blood, and different organs, including the bone marrow, and fat or adipose tissue. The term "adult" may be confusing because they are also found in fetal tissue. These cells are further developed than embryonic cells. The cell is considered adult, not the source. Adult stem cells, unlike embryonic stem cells, generally form cells in their own tissue type, making the chance of tumor formation unlikely. They also provide many types of growth factors that may stimulate the existing tissue to heal itself. The use of autologous stem cells precludes the necessity of immunosuppression when non-autologous cells are used.

There is now extensive evidence that bone marrow derived stem cells (BMSC) can regenerate non-hematopoietic tissues, including neural cells. Unlike embryonic stem cells, the use of BMSC avoids ethical issues. BMSC have been successfully used for many years to treat leukemia with bone marrow transplants.

J. N. Weiss, *Retinal and Optic Nerve Stem Cell Surgery*,
https://doi.org/10.1007/978-3-030-60850-7_1

Platelet-rich plasma (PRP) is the product of centrifuged whole blood with the red blood cells removed. It is an approximately 3–5 times physiologically concentrated source of growth factors, cytokines, and adult stem cells. The growth factors and cytokines include the following:

- Platelet-derived growth factor
- Transforming growth factor beta
- Fibroblast growth factor
- Insulin-like growth factor 1 and 2
- Vascular endothelial growth factor
- Epidermal growth factor
- Interleukin 8
- Keratinocyte growth factor
- Connective tissue growth factor

The platelets are activated by the thrombin and calcium chloride, which is used in preparation. Two PRP preparation methods have been approved by the US Food and Drug Administration (FDA). Anticoagulated whole blood undergoes a two-stage process of centrifugation in an FDA-approved, Class 2 device.

This treatment discussed in this book involves human cells and tissue (bone marrow derived stem cells or BMSC) and is exempt from IND requirements 21CFR312.2(b) and not subject to FDA oversight because it satisfies the following requirements:

(a) The material transferred is human cells, tissues, and cellular and tissue-based products (HCT/Ps) defined as "articles containing or consisting of human cells or tissues intended for implantation, transplantation, infusion or transfer into a human recipient" under 21 CFR 1261.3(d) (2011).
(b) The patient involved remains in the operating room during the entire surgical procedure, and the bone marrow and separated cells will remain in the same operating room as the patient during the entire procedure. This would exempt the procedure from FDA oversight as the exception set forth in Section 1271.15(b) "removing HCT/P's from an individual and implanting such HCT/P's into the same individual during the same surgical procedure."
(c) The HCT/Ps will undergo centrifugation only and therefore are considered minimally manipulated by FDA under 21 CRF 1271.10(a)(1). Specifically, "Minimal manipulation" is defined in 21 CFR 1271.3 (f) (2) as meaning "For cells or nonstructural tissues, processing that does not alter the relevant biological characteristics of cells or tissues."

In the preamble to the final HCT/P registration rule, the FDA listed several techniques that could be undertaken without causing tissues to be more than minimally manipulated including tissues that are centrifuged, subjected to density gradient separation, subjected to selective removal of a specific type of cell, sterilized or frozen.

In our protocols, the bone marrow aspirate is centrifuged in an FDA Class 2 device to provide separation of the stem cells satisfying the minimally manipulated criteria. There is no amplification or other interference with the function of the HCT/P. There is no drug used in the separation process. Furthermore, the device used for this centrifugation has complied with the regulatory processes and met the requirements of a Class 2 device per FDA guidelines, including minimal manipulation.

The material obtained is for homologous use only meeting the requirements of 21 CFR 1271.10(a) (2) which include the repair, reconstruction, replacement, or supplementation of a recipient's cells or tissues with HCT/P. The HCT/P is not being combined with a drug or device. Therefore, our technique is FDA compliant, and no "approval" is necessary.

In 2016, President Obama signed the 21st Century Cures Act, which provided an FDA provision for a Regenerative Medicine Advanced Therapy Designation (RMAT).

As described in Section 3033 of the 21st Century Cures Act, a drug is eligible for regenerative medicine advanced therapy (RMAT) designation if:

(a) "The drug is a regenerative medicine therapy, which is defined as a cell therapy, therapeutic tissue engineering product, human cell and tissue product, or any combination product using such therapies or products, except for those regulated solely under Section 361 of the Public Health Service Act and part 1271 of Title 21, Code of Federal Regulations;

(b) The drug is intended to treat, modify, reverse, or cure a serious or life-threatening disease or condition; and

(c) Preliminary clinical evidence indicates that the drug has the potential to address unmet medical needs for such disease or condition."

The Guidance for Industry Expedited Programs for Serious Conditions – Drugs and Biologics, section III.A., provides FDA's interpretation of whether a disease or condition is serious or life-threatening and whether a drug is intended to treat a serious disease or condition.

"The request for RMAT designation must be made either concurrently with submission of an Investigational New Drug application (IND) or as an amendment to an existing IND. We will not grant a RMAT designation if an IND is on hold or is placed on hold during the designation review.

We generally do not expect you to submit primary data (data sets), but your request for regenerative advanced therapy designation should describe the preliminary clinical evidence. Please include a brief description of any available therapies for the disease or condition, the study design, the population studied, and the endpoint(s) used; and a description of the study results and statistical analyses (e.g., subgroup analyses)."

Since our protocols are FDA compliant, and we are not using a drug, no IND is required; therefore, an RMAT designation is not applicable.

Chapter 2
History of Retinal Stem Cell Surgery

In 2009, I began my investigation of performing stem cell surgery for untreatable, potentially blinding, retina and optic nerve conditions. Following an extensive literature search, I located a clinic in Dusseldorf, Germany, that was performing retrobulbar injections of BMSC to treat age-related macular degeneration (AMD).

I visited the center several times and I performed the first subretinal placement of BMSC on two American patients at the center in 2010. One of the patients came to my office in the United States and was interviewed by a local television station. She had regained the ability to read a large-print book (YouTube – retinal stem cell surgery). In 2011, I performed the stem cell surgery on seven American patients in Vienna, Austria.

During this 2-year period, I was working on the stem cell surgery technique and mechanism, in consultation with ex-FDA attorneys, that would allow me to perform this procedure in the United States. I met with the FDA in 2011. I also visited/met with stem cell researchers from clinics in Mexico, Thailand, and Panama.

The stem cell clinic in Tijuana, Mexico, was using intravitreal injections of adipose-derived stem cells (ADSC) to treat age-related macular degeneration (AMD) with anecdotal good results. However, I examined a patient that had undergone the ADSC in Mexico that had developed proliferative vitreoretinopathy with a total retinal detachment, after receiving a subsequent intravitreal injection of Avastin for AMD. The pathology report of the vitreous specimen demonstrated adipose tissue. I also heard of complications in patients who received ADSC for ophthalmic conditions at other centers.

In 2016, three patients treated by a nurse in a Florida office with intravitreal ADSC lost their vision. The cases made national news and by innuendo, the supposed stem cell "experts" condemned all ocular stem cell procedures, because they were not "FDA approved." A true "expert" would have been familiar with the discussion above and not defame the researchers who were following the rules to the letter by performing FDA compliant research.

© The Author(s), under exclusive license to Springer Nature Switzerland AG 2021
J. N. Weiss, *Retinal and Optic Nerve Stem Cell Surgery*,
https://doi.org/10.1007/978-3-030-60850-7_2

Of note, FDA regulations technically do not allow the use of ADSC for medical treatments outside of their approval. The FDA has ruled that the processing of the adipose tissue to isolate the stem cells is more than the "minimal manipulation" allowed by their regulations.

Chapter 3
Funding

Unless you are independently wealthy and a philanthropist, someone must pay you to work. At the end of the day, you can have all the good intentions and empathy in the world, but you must eat, wear clothes, have a place to live, and if you have a family, support them as well. Nothing can be accomplished in science, or in life, without money. Rent, equipment, supplies, personnel, etc., must all be paid for.

A clinical trial, also called an interventional trial, is a type of research where participants receive a specific intervention that is dictated by a study protocol. The intervention may be a surgical procedure, drug, device, or a change to the participants' behavior, such as a diet. Clinical trials may compare a new medical or surgical approach to no intervention. There are various sources that provide funding for clinical trials.

The National Institutes of Health (NIH)

The NIH is the largest biomedical funding source in the United States. There has been a 20% inflation adjusted decline in the NIH budget over the last decade. Approximately 15–20% of grant submissions receive funding, and due to government budget sequestration, investigators receive only 90% of the approved funds. A 2007 US government study found that university faculty members spend approximately 40% of their research time navigating bureaucracy in order to receive funding for their work.

A research grant is awarded to an individual at a university, but not to the same individual when he enters private practice, effectively removing an experienced researcher from government funding. NIH grants are typically for a 3-year period and end abruptly if not renewed. In addition, the researcher is unable to shift the funds to another project if the first project is not successful.

© The Author(s), under exclusive license to Springer Nature Switzerland AG 2021   7
J. N. Weiss, *Retinal and Optic Nerve Stem Cell Surgery*,
https://doi.org/10.1007/978-3-030-60850-7_3

Pharmaceutical Companies

Pharmaceutical companies are commercial enterprises organized to make money. Approximately 75% of clinical trials in medicine are company sponsored. Such funding may introduce bias, as the study design or interpretation is more likely to favor the drug under consideration with the ultimate goal, the attainment of FDA approval. This is understandable as the time to develop a successful drug is 10–15 years, and the cost to achieve FDA approval has successively increased over the decades to approximately 1.2 billion dollars at the present time.

An orphan disease is defined as any disease affecting up to 200,000 individuals in the United States. There are incentives offered to pharmaceutical companies through the Orphan Drug Act of 1983 to address the rare disease market. However, orphan diseases with larger numbers of patients or those diseases for which there may be less price resistance regarding any successful treatment may draw development efforts in an unfair way.

Nonprofit Organizations

Like the NIH, nonprofit organizations use a panel of experts who decide the worthiness of a particular grant and determine the awarding of funding. As such, they suffer from the same problem as the NIH.

Thomas Kuhn has pointed out that breakthrough insights frequently stem from the intersection of disciplines, not from within the discipline. Grant reviewers are generally within the same discipline and do not recognize the new paradigm that may have come from the work of scientists in other fields. They remain committed to the old paradigm that has shaped their beliefs, which prompted the physicist, Max Planck, to say, "New scientific truth does not triumph by convincing its opponents and making them see the light, but rather because its opponents eventually die, and a new generation grows up that is familiar with it." Also like the NIH, nonprofit organizations award grants to institutions, not to individual researchers in private practice.

Private-Funded Research

This includes a broad pool of donors with a wide range of passions that may speed progress by investing in bold ideas, gambles, and risky projects. Decisions may be made quickly, not encumbered by large bureaucracies. A sense of urgency can be respected.

Critics argue that gifts privatize research and steer resources toward areas of personal interest. Supporters argue that it is the personal choice of the funder whether money is spent on personal goods or personal research. Personally funded projects have a vested interest in solving the chosen problem and, unlike pharmaceutically funded research, are not subject to the profit motive or market forces.

Patient-Funded Foundations

It is not uncommon for many patients with rare diseases or their families to set up support groups, particularly with the ready availability of social networking. In some cases, the only research foundations focused on particularly rare diseases have been initiated by patients and families affected by those diseases. There are over 7000 rare genetic diseases impacting 8–10% of the US population or about 25 million patients. When such a disease afflicts a high profile or financially successful individual, or their family member, that particular disease can receive disproportionate attention and support.

Patient-Funded Research

In this model, the patient pays for participating in the clinical research. In terms of the research, this is similar to the private-funded model discussed above. Less common conditions and risky proposals may be studied, unencumbered by bureaucracy, and coupled with the ability to make quick decisions.

Critics argue that desperate patients can be exploited and should not pay for clinical research. Clearly, people with resources decide how to use their resources. Not allowing patients to pay for research would restrict their ability to use their own resources as they see fit.

Unlike other types of funding, patient-funded research is subject to market demands. If a study is too expensive, there will be less participants, unlike the situation where the funding is provided for the patient to participate in the research. The self-funding patient will be more inclined to demand information thus providing a more thought-out informed consent than in a study where free care is provided, as they want to receive their "money's worth." One can argue that free medical care may be considered an exploitative inducement to participate in research.

Patient-funded studies are generally for conditions not being investigated by NIH, or pharmaceutical studies, and tend toward novel approaches for less prevalent medical problems.

Patient-funded research has been criticized for, by its nature, it eliminates the participation of individuals who cannot afford to participate. One can make the same criticism for the other funding sources as unless the study pays the patient for participation, including travel costs, individuals may be unable to take the required time off from work, nor have the financial and personal support structure in place to engage in a study.

Since the purpose of a research study is to determine whether the clinical intervention is of benefit, and such interventions may carry some medical risk, one could argue that aligning financial cost with participation creates a higher level of patient engagement, risk benefit assessment, and therefore informed consent. In addition, the ultimate benefits of basic and clinical research accrue to all individuals with a particular disease irrespective of financial wherewithal.

Does profit taint the research? One could argue that all human activity creates bias; otherwise, there would be no activity. Unless the research is self-funded, researchers are always paid by some funding source; otherwise, they could not perform the research.

Frequently, both NIH and pharmaceutical funding are proportional to the number of subjects the researcher enrolls in the study, which some may consider to be unethical. In this respect, the patient-funded study differs little from other types of studies. As pointed out previously, it is in the researcher's interest to keep the patient cost at a reasonable level in order to encourage patient entry.

The patient-funded study, which has a detailed protocol, has undergone Institutional Review Board review, is listed with ClinicalTrials.gov (NIH), is collecting data, and is publishing results, whether positive or negative, is an important form of research allowing the testing of ideas that would otherwise languish due to a lack of funding.

All human endeavors require work and effort and therefore have financial costs. There is a range of how removed the patients are from those costs, depending on the research payment methodology.

In the case of publicly funded clinical research, the patient may have low awareness of the cost of the clinical research as the funds are taken from the general tax base of whose allocation individuals have minimal awareness. In publicly funded research, the cost of an individual's participation is spread out over millions of people, and therefore the percentage of cost that is the responsibility of an individual patient is low. This low awareness of source and percentage cost of participation removes these particular financial considerations from the informed consent process.

On the other end of the spectrum, patient-funded research causes high awareness of the cost of that individual's participation and causes a high percentage of the cost to be the responsibility of the participating patient. This high awareness enters the informed consent process as an additional consideration as patients weigh the potential personal benefit of participation. This causes a pause in this process, even for the wealthiest individuals.

Pharmaceutical clinical research would fall in-between, with the actual costs being deferred to a later time, but still assumed by the individual patient needing the successfully proven care depending on the health insurance methodology.

   In considering the different methods of funding of clinical research, the overall benefit of properly done clinical research, from whichever funding source, should be kept in mind. All clinical research and patient care creates costs, which ultimately accrue to individuals in the society. It is only a matter of how directly those costs are felt by individuals. Unlike grants, with time-limited support, patient-funded studies may be self-perpetuating. As long as the public perceives benefit, the study may continue.

Chapter 4
ClinicalTrials.gov Listings

In the first three chapters, I have provided the scientific and regulatory basis for this work, the history, and the rationale for a patient-funded study. Decades after stem cells were discovered, the Stem Cell Ophthalmology Trial remains the only avenue for patients with "untreatable" retinal and optic nerve conditions.

In the next sections, I will describe the mechanisms by which a clinical study may be performed. Provided is our listing on www.ClinicalTrials.gov, our protocols, study design, informed consent, and additional patient explanation.

Photographs of the various postoperative stages of each surgical procedure are presented as are thoughts for the future. For those that are interested, there is a listing of our publications and answers to the most "frequently asked questions."

The Stem Cell Ophthalmology Treatment Study (SCOTS) is an Institutional Board Approved Study registered with NIH. ClinicalTrials.gov Identifier: NCT01920867. Here is the listing of SCOTS 1 on the NIH website. When SCOTS 1 fulfilled its enrollment (300 patients) the study ended, and SCOTS 2 began. The SCOTS 2 listing follows. Only pertinent information is provided.

SCOTS I

- Stem Cell Ophthalmology Treatment Study (SCOTS)
- ClinicalTrials.gov Identifier: NCT01920867

Purpose

This study will evaluate the use of autologous bone marrow derived stem cells (BMSC) for the treatment of retinal and optic nerve damage or disease.

© The Author(s), under exclusive license to Springer Nature Switzerland AG 2021
J. N. Weiss, *Retinal and Optic Nerve Stem Cell Surgery*,
https://doi.org/10.1007/978-3-030-60850-7_4

Condition:
- Retinal Disease Procedure: RB (Retrobulbar)
- Procedure: ST (Subtenon)
- Procedure: IV (Intravenous)
- Procedure: IVIT (Intravitreal)
- Procedure: IO (Intraocular)
- Macular Degeneration
- Hereditary Retinal Dystrophy
- Optic Nerve Disease
- Glaucoma

Study Type:
- Interventional

Study Design:
- Allocation: Non-Randomized
- Endpoint Classification: Efficacy Study
- Intervention Model: Parallel Assignment
- Masking: Open Label
- Primary Purpose: Treatment

Official Title:
- Bone Marrow Derived Stem Cell Ophthalmology Treatment Study

Primary Outcome Measures:

1. Visual acuity [Time Frame: 1 day to 12 months] [Designated as safety issue: No] Best corrected visual acuity will be measured with Snellen Eye Chart and the ETDRS (Early Treatment Diabetic Retinopathy Study) Eye Chart when available at each post-procedure visit. Intervals at minimum will be first post-procedure day, then 3 months, 6 months, and 12 months post-procedure day. Recommended visit 1-month post-procedure day.

Secondary Outcome Measures:

1. Visual fields [Time Frame: 1 day to 12 months] [Designated as safety issue: No] Visual fields will be evaluated with automated perimetry during post-procedure visits as needed and specifically at 6 months and 12 months.

Estimated Enrollment:
- 300
- Study Start Date: August 2013

Estimated Study Completion Date:
- August 2017

Estimated Primary Completion Date:
- August 2016 (Final data collection date for primary outcome measure)

- Arms
- Assigned Interventions
- Active Comparator: RB, ST, IV
- Injections of BMSC retrobulbar (RB), subtenon (ST), and intravenous (IV)

- Procedure: RB (Retrobulbar)
- Retrobulbar injection of Bone Marrow Derived Stem
- Cells (BMSC)
- Other Name: Retrobulbar injection of stem cells

- Procedure: ST (Subtenon)
- Subtenon injection of Bone Marrow Derived Stem
- Cells (BMSC)
- Other Name: Subtenon injection of stem cells

- Procedure: IV (Intravenous)
- Intravenous injection of Bone Marrow Derived Stem
- Cells (BMSC)

- Procedure: IVIT (Intravitreal)
- Intravitreal injection of Bone Marrow Derived Stem
- Cells (BMSC)
- Other Name: Intravitreal injection of stem cells
- Active Comparator: RB, ST, IV, IO
- Injection of BMSC retrobulbar, subtenon, intravenous, and intraocular (IO) with vitrectomy

- Procedure: IO (Intraocular)
- Intraocular injection of Bone Marrow Derived Stem
- Cells (BMSC) with vitrectomy prior to intraocular injection. For example, may include larger amount of stem cells in the intravitreal cavity, intraneuronal injections, or subretinal injections of stem cells
- Other Name: Intraocular injection of stem cells with vitrectomy

Detailed Description

Eyes with loss of vision from retinal or optic nerve conditions generally considered irreversible will be treated with a combination of injections of autologous bone marrow derived stem cells isolated from the bone marrow using standard medical and surgical practices.

Retinal conditions may include degenerative, ischemic, or physical damage (examples may include macular degeneration, hereditary retinal dystrophies such as retinitis pigmentosa, Stargardt disease, non-perfusion retinopathies, post retinal detachment).

Optic nerve conditions may include degenerative, ischemic, or physical damage (examples may include optic nerve damage from glaucoma, compression, ischemic optic neuropathy, optic atrophy). Injections may include retrobulbar, subtenon, intravitreal, intraocular, subretinal, and intravenous. Patients will be followed for 12 months with serial comprehensive eye examinations including relevant imaging and diagnostic ophthalmic testing.

Eligibility

Ages Eligible for Study:
• 18 Years and older (Adult, Senior)

Genders Eligible for Study:
• Both

Accepts Healthy Volunteers:
• No

Criteria

• Inclusion Criteria:

1. Have objective, documented damage to the retina or optic nerve unlikely to improve.
2. Have objective, documented damage to the retina or optic nerve that is progressive.
3. Have less than or equal to 20/40 best corrected central visual acuity in one or both eyes *and/or* an abnormal visual field in one or both eyes.
4. Be at least 3 months post-surgical treatment intended to treat any ophthalmologic disease and stable.
5. If under current medical therapy (pharmacologic treatment) for a retinal or optic nerve disease be considered stable on that treatment and unlikely to have visual function improvement (e.g., glaucoma with intraocular pressure stable on topical medications but visual field damage).
6. Have the potential for improvement with BMSC treatment and be at minimal risk of any potential harm from the procedure.
7. Be over the age of 18.
8. Be medically stable and able to be medically cleared by their primary care physician or a licensed primary care practitioner for the procedure. Medical

clearance means that in the estimation of the primary care practitioner, the patient can reasonably be expected to undergo the procedure without significant medical risk to health.

- Exclusion Criteria:
  1. Patients who are not capable of an adequate ophthalmologic examination or evaluation to document the pathology.
  2. Patients who are not capable or not willing to undergo follow-up eye exams with the Principal Investigator or their ophthalmologist or optometrist as outlined in the protocol.
  3. Patients who are not capable of providing informed consent.
  4. Patients who may be at significant risk to general health or to the eyes and visual function should they undergo the procedure.

Contacts and Locations

Choosing to participate in a study is an important personal decision. Talk with your doctor and family members or friends about deciding to join a study. To learn more about this study, you or your doctor may contact the study research staff using the Contacts provided below. For general information, see Learn About Clinical Studies.

Please refer to this study by its ClinicalTrials.gov identifier: NCT01920867

Contacts
- Contact: Steven Levy, MD
- 203-423-9494
- stevenlevy@mdstemcells.com

- Principal Investigator: Jeffrey Weiss, MD
- Sub-Investigator: Steven Levy, MD
- United Arab Emirates

- Recruiting
- Dubai, United Arab Emirates

Responsible Party:
- Retina Associates of South Florida

ClinicalTrials.gov Identifier:
- NCT01920867 History of Changes

Other Study ID Numbers:
- ICMS-2013-0019.

Keywords Provided by Retina Associates of South Florida:
- Stem Cells
- Dry Macular Degeneration
- Wet Macular Degeneration
- Retinal Atrophy
- Retinal Dystrophy
- Hereditary Retinal Dystrophy
- Retinitis Pigmentosa
- Stargardt Disease
- Cone Dystrophy
- Cone-Rod Dystrophy
- Maculopathy
- Optic Nerve Disease
- Optic Nerve Atrophy
- Optic Atrophy
- Ischemic Optic Neuropathy
- Bone Marrow Derived Stem Cells
- BMSC
- BMC (Bone Marrow Cell)
- Mesenchymal Stem Cells
- MSC
- Eye Disease
- Eye Stem Cells
- Ophthalmology
- Ophthalmic Disease
- Retina
- Retinal Disease
- Macular Degeneration
- Age-Related Macular Degeneration
- Myopic Macular Degeneration
- Glaucoma
- Ocular Hypertension
- Eye Diseases
- Retinal Degeneration
- Cranial Nerve Diseases
- Macular Degeneration
- Retinal Diseases
- Retinal Dystrophies
- Nervous System Diseases

Once we treated the 300 patients authorized in SCOTS 1, SCOTS 2, which allows the treatment of 500 patients, began. This is the current study.

Stem Cell Ophthalmology Treatment Study II (SCOTS2)

This study is currently recruiting participants.

- MD Stem Cells
- ClinicalTrials.gov Identifier: NCT03011541

Purpose

This study will evaluate the use of autologous bone marrow derived stem cells (BMSC) for the treatment of retinal and optic nerve damage or disease.

- Condition
- Intervention
- Retinal Disease
- Age-Related Macular Degeneration
- Retinitis Pigmentosa
- Stargardt Disease
- Optic Neuropathy
- Nonarteritic Ischemic Optic Neuropathy
- Optic Atrophy
- Optic Nerve Disease
- Glaucoma
- Leber Hereditary Optic Neuropathy

- Procedure: Arm 1
- Procedure: Arm 2
- Procedure: Arm 3

Study Type:
- Interventional

Study Design:
- Allocation: Non-Randomized
- Intervention Model: Parallel Assignment
- Masking: None (Open Label)
- Primary Purpose: Treatment

Official Title:
• Bone Marrow Derived Stem Cell Ophthalmology Treatment Study II

Primary Outcome Measures:
• Visual Acuity [Time Frame: Change from pre-procedure to 12 months] Best cor-rected visual acuity will be measured with Snellen Eye Chart and the ETDRS (Early Treatment Diabetic Retinopathy Study) Eye Chart when available at each post-procedure visit. Intervals at minimum will be first post-procedure day, then 3 months, 6 months, and 12 months post-procedure day. Recommended visit 1-month post-procedure day.

Secondary Outcome Measures:
• Visual Fields [Time Frame: Change from pre-procedure to 12 months] Visual fields will be evaluated with automated perimetry during post-procedure visits as needed and specifically at 6 months and 12 months. Visual fields are a key mea-surement in patients with peripheral vision loss.
• Optical Coherence Tomography (OCT) [Time Frame: Change from pre-procedure to 12 months] OCT thickness of the retinal nerve fiber layer the optic nerve and/or macula during the post-procedure visits as needed and specifically at 6 and 12 months – if available.

Estimated Enrollment:
• 500

Study Start Date:
• January 2016

Estimated Study Completion Date:
• January 2021

Estimated Primary Completion Date:
• January 2020 (Final data collection date for primary outcome measure)

• Arms
• Assigned Interventions
• Active Comparator: Arm 1
• BMSC provided retrobulbar, subtenon, and intravenous for one or both eyes

• Procedure: Arm 1
• Procedure/Surgery: RB (Retrobulbar)
• Retrobulbar injection of Bone Marrow Derived Stem Cells (BMSC)

• Procedure/Surgery: ST (Subtenon)
• Subtenon injection of Bone Marrow Derived Stem Cells (BMSC)
• Procedure/Surgery: IV (Intravenous)
• Intravenous injection of Bone Marrow Derived Stem Cells (BMSC)

Other Names:
- Retrobulbar (RB)
- Subtenon (ST)
- Intravenous (IV)

- Active Comparator: Arm 2
- BMSC provided retrobulbar, subtenon, intravitreal, and intravenous for one or both eyes.

- Procedure: Arm 2

- Procedure/Surgery: RB (Retrobulbar)
- Retrobulbar injection of Bone Marrow Derived Stem Cells (BMSC)

- Procedure/Surgery: ST (Subtenon)
- Subtenon injection of Bone Marrow Derived Stem Cells (BMSC)

- Procedure/Surgery: IV (Intravenous)
- Intravenous injection of Bone Marrow Derived Stem Cells (BMSC)

- Procedure/Surgery: IVIT (Intravitreal)
- Intravitreal injection of Bone Marrow Derived Stem Cells (BMSC)

- Active Comparator: Arm 3
- BMSC provided either intra-optic nerve or subretinal for eye with worse vision with fellow eye receiving either retrobulbar and subtenon or retrobulbar, subtenon, and intravitreal; followed by intravenous.

- Procedure: Arm 1
- Procedure/Surgery: RB (Retrobulbar)
- Retrobulbar injection of Bone Marrow Derived Stem Cells (BMSC)

- Procedure/Surgery: ST (Subtenon)
- Subtenon injection of Bone Marrow Derived Stem Cells (BMSC)

- Procedure/Surgery: IV (Intravenous)
- Intravenous injection of Bone Marrow Derived Stem Cells (BMSC)

- Procedure: Arm 2
- Procedure/Surgery: RB (Retrobulbar)
- Retrobulbar injection of Bone Marrow Derived Stem Cells (BMSC)

- Procedure/Surgery: ST (Subtenon)
- Subtenon injection of Bone Marrow Derived Stem Cells (BMSC)

- Procedure/Surgery: IV (Intravenous)
- Intravenous injection of Bone Marrow Derived Stem Cells (BMSC)

- Procedure/Surgery: IVIT (Intravitreal)
- Intravitreal injection of Bone Marrow Derived Stem Cells (BMSC)

- Procedure: Arm 3
- Procedure/Surgery: RB (Retrobulbar)
- Retrobulbar injection of Bone Marrow Derived Stem Cells (BMSC)
- Procedure/Surgery: ST (Subtenon)
- Subtenon injection of Bone Marrow Derived Stem Cells (BMSC)

- Procedure/Surgery: IV (Intravenous)
- Intravenous injection of Bone Marrow Derived Stem Cells (BMSC)
- Procedure/Surgery: IO (Intraocular)
- Intraocular injection of Bone Marrow Derived Stem Cells (BMSC) with vitrectomy prior to intraocular injection. For example, may include larger amount of stem cells in the intravitreal cavity, intraneuronal injections or subretinal injections of stem cells.

Detailed Description

Eyes with loss of vision from retinal or optic nerve conditions generally considered irreversible will be treated with a combination of injections of autologous bone marrow derived stem cells isolated from the bone marrow using standard medical and surgical practices. Retinal conditions may include degenerative, ischemic, or physical damage (examples may include macular degeneration, hereditary retinal dystrophies such as retinitis pigmentosa, Stargardt disease, non-perfusion retinopathies, post retinal detachment).

Optic nerve conditions may include degenerative, ischemic, or physical damage (examples may include optic nerve damage from glaucoma, compression, ischemic optic neuropathy, optic atrophy). Injections may include retrobulbar, subtenon, intravitreal, intraocular, subretinal, and intravenous. Patients will be followed for 12 months with serial comprehensive eye examinations including relevant imaging and diagnostic ophthalmic testing.

Eligibility

Ages Eligible for Study:
- 18 Years and older (Adult, Senior)

Sexes Eligible for Study:
- All

Accepts Healthy Volunteers:
- No

Criteria

Inclusion Criteria:
- Have objective, documented damage to the retina or optic nerve unlikely to improve.
- Have objective, documented damage to the retina or optic nerve that is progressive *and* have less than or equal to 20/40 best corrected central visual acuity in one or both eyes *and/or* an abnormal visual field in one or both eyes.
- Be at least 3 months post-surgical treatment intended to treat any ophthalmologic disease and is stable.
- If under current medical therapy (pharmacologic treatment) for a retinal or optic nerve disease be considered stable on that treatment and unlikely to have visual function improvement (e.g., glaucoma with intraocular pressure stable on topical medications but visual field damage).
- Have the potential for improvement with BMSC treatment and be at minimal risk of any potential harm from the procedure.
- Be over the age of 18.
- Be medically stable and able to be medically cleared by their primary care physician or a licensed primary care practitioner for the procedure.
- Medical clearance means that in the estimation of the primary care practitioner, the patient can reasonably be expected to undergo the procedure without significant medical risk to health.

Exclusion Criteria:
- Patients who are not capable of an adequate ophthalmologic examination or evaluation to document the pathology.
- Patients who are not capable or not willing to undergo follow-up eye exams with the Principal Investigator or their ophthalmologist or optometrist as outlined in the protocol.
- Patients who are not capable of providing informed consent.
- Patients who may be at significant risk to general health or to the eyes and visual function should they undergo the procedure.

Contacts and Locations

Choosing to participate in a study is an important personal decision. Talk with your doctor and family members or friends about deciding to join a study. To learn more about this study, you or your doctor may contact the study research staff using the Contacts provided below. For general information, see Learn About Clinical Studies.

Please refer to this study by its ClinicalTrials.gov identifier: NCT03011541

Contacts
- Contact: Steven Levy, MD
- 203-423-9494
- stevenlevy@mdstemcells.com

Locations
- United States, Florida
- The Healing Institute
- Recruiting
- Margate, Florida, United States, 33063
- Contact: Steven Levy, MD 203-423-9494 stevenlevy@mdstemcells.com
- Principal Investigator: Jeffrey N Weiss, MD
- United Arab Emirates
- Enrolling by invitation
- Dubai, United Arab Emirates
- Sponsors and Collaborators
- MD Stem Cells
- Investigators
- Study Director:
- Steven Levy, MD
- MD Stem Cells
- Principal Investigator:
- Jeffrey N. Weiss, MD
- The Healing Institute

More Information

Additional Information:
- Seeing is Believing: South Florida Doctor Helps the Blind See Through Experimental Procedure
- Baltimore woman once blind, regains vision after retinal stem cell surgery (see link, website, clinicaltrials.gov).

Responsible Party:
- MD Stem Cells
- ClinicalTrials.gov Identifier:
- NCT03011541 History of Changes

Other Study ID Numbers:
- SCOTS2

Study First Received:
- January 1, 2017

Last Updated:
- July 17, 2017

Keywords Provided by MD Stem Cells:
- Stem Cells
- Bone Marrow Derived Stem Cells
- BMSC
- Mesenchymal Stem Cells
- MSC
- Eye Disease
- Ophthalmology
- Ophthalmic Disease
- Retina
- Retinal Disease
- Macular Degeneration
- Age-Related Macular Degeneration
- Myopic Macular Degeneration
- Geographic Atrophy
- Dry Macular Degeneration
- Wet Macular Degeneration
- Retinal Atrophy
- Retinal Dystrophy
- Hereditary Retinal Dystrophy
- Malattia Leventinese
- Retinitis Pigmentosa
- Stargardt Disease
- Cone Dystrophy
- Rod-Cone Dystrophy
- Cone-Rod Dystrophy
- Maculopathy
- Optic Nerve Disease
- Optic Atrophy

- Optic Neuropathy
- Ischemic Optic Neuropathy
- Additional relevant MeSH terms:
- Peripheral Nervous System Diseases
- Macular Degeneration
- Atrophy
- Retinitis
- Retinitis Pigmentosa
- Optic Nerve Diseases
- Retinal Diseases
- Optic Neuropathy, Ischemic
- Optic Atrophy, Hereditary, Leber
- Nervous System Diseases
- Optic Atrophy
- Neuromuscular Diseases
- Retinal Degeneration
- Eye Diseases
- Pathological Conditions, Anatomical
- Eye Diseases, Hereditary
- Retinal Dystrophies
- Genetic Diseases, Inborn
- Cranial Nerve Diseases
- Vascular Diseases
- Cardiovascular Diseases
- Optic Atrophies, Hereditary
- Heredodegenerative Disorders, Nervous System
- Neurodegenerative Diseases
- Mitochondrial Diseases
- Metabolic Diseases

Institutional Review Board approval in the United States is limited to those patient 18 years of age and older. We are able to treat patients younger than 18 years of age at Fakeeh University Hospital, in Dubai. This is a modern, state-of-the art hospital with excellent support services. The hospital is approved by the US Joint Commission on Accreditation.

Chapter 5
Study Protocols

- Study Protocols (submitted to the IRB). I have included the most recent, SCOTS 2 protocol.
- Protocol Title:
- Bone Marrow Derived Stem Cell Ophthalmology Treatment Study II

- Protocol Number: 2
- Date of Protocol: October 23, 2015

- Working Title: SCOTS II
- Sponsor and Principal Investigator:
- Jeffrey N. Weiss, MD
- Retina Associates of South Florida
- 5800 Colonial Drive, Suite 300
- Margate, FL 33063
- Telephone 954-975-0044

- Sub-Investigator:
- Steven Levy MD
- MD Stem Cells
- 412 Main Street, Suite I
- Ridgefield, CT 06877
- Telephone 203-423-9494

- Primary Site:
- Retina Associates of South Florida
- 5800 Colonial Drive, Suite 300
- Margate, FL 33063
- Telephone 954-975-0044

J. N. Weiss, *Retinal and Optic Nerve Stem Cell Surgery*,
https://doi.org/10.1007/978-3-030-60850-7_5

- Supplemental Site:
- Park Creek Surgery Center
- 6806 North State Road 7
- Coconut Creek, Florida 33073

Introduction

Type of Research

This is a human clinical study involving the isolation of autologous bone marrow derived stem cells (BMSC) and its transfer to the eyes via retrobulbar, subtenon, intraocular, and intravenous in order to determine if such a treatment will provide a statistically significant improvement in visual function for patients with retinal and optic nerve eye disease or damage. BMSC are predominately CD34 and are considered by investigators to be pluripotent. In this study, we will be providing a transfer of these pluripotent stem cells from the bone marrow where they predominately reside to damaged retinal and optic nerve tissue.

This research is not federally funded nor subject to federal oversight. There is no HDE involved.

This treatment involves human cells and tissue (bone marrow derived stem cells or BMSC) and is exempt from IND requirement 21CFR312.2(b) and not subject to FDA oversight because it satisfies the following requirements:

1. The material transferred is human cells, tissues, and cellular and tissue based products (HCT/Ps) defined as "articles containing or consisting of human cells or tissues intended for implantation, transplantation, infusion or transfer into a human recipient" under 21 CFR 1261.3(d) (2011).
2. The patient remains in the operating room during the entire surgical procedure, and the bone marrow and separated cells will remain in the same operating room as the patient during the entire procedure. This would exempt the procedure from FDA oversight as the exception set forth in Section 1271.15(b) "removing HCT/P's from an individual and implanting such HCT/P's into the same individual during the same surgical procedure."
3. The HCT/Ps will undergo centrifugation only and therefore are considered minimally manipulated by FDA under 21 CRF 1271.10(a)(1). Specifically, "Minimal manipulation" is defined in 21 CFR 1271.3 (f) (2) as meaning "For cells or nonstructural tissues, processing that does not alter the relevant biological characteristics of cells or tissues." In the preamble to the final HCT/P registration rule, FDA listed several techniques that could be undertaken without causing tissues to be more than minimally manipulated including tissues that are centrifuged, subjected to density gradient separation, subjected to selective removal of a specific type of cell, sterilized or frozen.

In our protocol, the bone marrow tissue will be centrifuged in an FDA Class 2 device to provide separation of the stem cells satisfying the minimally manipulated criteria. There will be no amplification or other interference with the function of the HCT/P. There is no drug used in the separation process. Furthermore, the device used for this centrifugation has complied with the regulatory processes and met the requirements of a Class 2 device per FDA guidelines, including minimal manipulation.

4. The material obtained is for homologous use only meeting the requirements of 21 CFR 1271.10(a) (2) which includes the repair, reconstruction, replacement, or supplementation of a recipient's cells or tissues with HCT/P. We believe that bone marrow derived stem cells function in the same fashion no matter their location.
5. The HCT/P is not being combined with a drug or device.

Purpose and Objective of the Study

The purpose of the study is to continue to evaluate the use of autologous bone marrow derived stem cells for retinal and optic nerve tissue damage and determine whether they will show a statistically significant improvement in visual function for progressive and otherwise untreatable retinal and optic nerve eye disease or damage. The objective is to determine which diseases or injuries of the retina and optic nerve and at what stages they may be most effectively treated.

Background of the Study

Rationale for SCOTS II

The original Bone Marrow Derived Stem Cell Ophthalmology Study or SCOTS is being successfully conducted but will reach the limit of its enrollment soon. This study has been very successful in establishing the safety and efficacy of bone marrow derived stem cells (BMSC) in a number of retinal and optic nerve diseases. The study has begun publishing and will continue to publish based on the data from patients who have undergone treatment. However, there has been variability in demographics of the patients including age, length of disease process, visual acuity, comorbidities, and the fact that many of the patients have had a mixture of retinal and/or optic nerve diseases.

In addition, the need to continue establishing the value of BMSC treatment for the medical community remains. Medicine is traditionally very slow to adopt new procedures and approaches to treatment. Physicians and the healthcare industry typically require multiple studies and continuing effort to explore and establish procedures. Therefore, it remains our goal to continue treating patients within an IRB approved protocol, which will allow publishing of results in reputable medical journals. SCOTS II will allow us to continue recruiting patients and to increase the numbers of more closely matched demographics within specific diseases.

Current Publications

(See Chap. 11)

Background Information Regarding Original SCOTS (ICMS-2013-0019)

The clinical use of stem cells has been ongoing for several years now in many parts of the world. It is estimated that over 20,000 patients have undergone stem cell therapies of one type or another with variable improvements in their disease conditions.

Sources for these stem cells have included umbilical cord, fetal, adipose, placental, and bone marrow. Depending on the country and regulatory environment, there has been variation in the scientific reliability of these treatments. However, the continued anecdotal reports of subjective improvements in many conditions and testimonials on the part of individuals with progressive or untreatable diseases provide encouragement for patients to seek out these treatments.

The use of bone marrow derived material in orthopedics for enhancement of healing, joint treatment, and other orthopedic procedures is well established in the United States. Bone marrow derived stem cells have also been used in patients with a variety of diseases including neurologic, cardiac, immunologic, degenerative, and ophthalmic. Clinics in Germany, Austria, Thailand, Mexico, China, and other countries have treated patients with various eye diseases with stem cells and anecdotal results have been encouraging. The continuing complaint within the medical community in the United States is a lack of objective, scientifically verified results. Therefore, ophthalmologic stem cell treatments in the United States remain marginalized, and patients and their physicians remain confused as to its value.

The time has come to provide a solid study of the effects of BMSC on damaged retinal and optic nerve tissue and the variety of progressive eye disease responsible for that damage. This will help establish which diseases are most likely to benefit and at what stages they are likely to benefit in order to provide guidelines for treatment.

Participant Selection

A. Inclusion and Exclusion Criteria

- Inclusions:

The treatment with BMSC is a tissue transfer of active, predominately CD34 stem cells from the bone marrow to the tissues surrounding or within the eye for the purpose of improving function of that tissue. Diminished visual acuity (central vision or what the patient can read on the eye chart) and reduced peripheral vision (vision to the side) can occur as a result of progressive damage to the retina or optic nerve from disease or injury.

The exact disease or injury process causing the damage may vary, but the end result may be damage to photoreceptors of the retina; to the support cells of the photoreceptors called the RPE/retinal pigment epithelium; to the inner or outer plexiform layer of retinal neurons; to the nerve fiber layer forming the optic nerve either within the retina to the ganglion cell bodies/axons or of the ganglion cell axons or glial support cells within the optic nerve proper; or to the vascular supply of any of these tissues. It is important to understand that our treatment protocol relates to transferring cells from one part of the body (bone marrow) in a way that will maximize the damaged tissue's access to those cells in a safe and reasonable fashion. There are many diseases and injuries that cause progressive damage to these tissues. Our goal is treatment of the damaged tissue rather than a specific disease. To be eligible for treatment patients must:

1. Have objective, documented damage to the retina or optic nerve unlikely to improve.
2. Have objective, documented damage to the retina or optic nerve that is progressive
3. Have less than or equal to 20/40 central visual acuity in one or both eyes *and/or* an abnormal visual field in one or both eyes.
4. Be at least 3 months post-surgical treatment intended to treat any ophthalmologic disease and is stable.
5. If under current medical therapy (pharmacologic treatment) for a retinal or optic nerve disease be considered stable on that treatment and unlikely to have visual function improvement (e.g., glaucoma with intraocular pressure stable on topical medications but visual field damage).

6. Have the potential for improvement with BMSC treatment and be at minimal risk of any potential harm from the procedure.
7. Have no alternative treatment that could improve their visual function at the stage of disease presenting.
8. Be over the age of 18.
9. Be medically stable and able to be medically cleared by their primary care physician or a licensed primary care practitioner for the procedure. Medical clearance means that in the estimation of the primary care practitioner, the patient can reasonably be expected to undergo the procedure without significant medical risk to health.

– Restrictions:

1. All patients must be capable of an adequate retinal examination and evaluation to document the pathology. This will include the ability to cooperate with the exam, sufficiently clear media (cornea, lens, vitreous), and sufficient pupillary dilation.
2. Patients must be capable and willing to undergo follow-up eye examinations with Dr. Weiss or their ophthalmologist or optometrist as outlined in the protocol.
3. Patients must be capable of providing informed consent.
4. In the estimation of Dr. Weiss, the BMSC collection and eye treatment will not present a significant risk of harm to the patient's general health or to the eyes and visual function.
5. Patients with retinal or optic nerve damage actively undergoing treatment providing the potential for improvement in visual function will not be eligible. At least 3 months must have elapsed following any treatment for non-posterior disease (e.g., cataract surgery) or posterior segment disease (e.g., laser photocoagulation or intravitreal injection of VEGF inhibitors for wet macular degeneration) before the patient may be eligible.
6. Patients who are not medically stable or who may be at significant risk to their health undergoing the procedure will not be eligible.
7. Women of childbearing age must not be pregnant at the time of treatment and should refrain from becoming pregnant for 3 months post treatment.

B. Gender – no restrictions. Women of child bearing age are eligible, but must not be pregnant at the time of treatment.
C. Racial/ethnic origin – no restrictions.
D. Vulnerable populations – no vulnerable populations will be eligible.
E. Age – no patients under the age of 18 are to be enrolled. For those 18 years and older, there are no age restrictions.
F. Total number of participants to be enrolled: 500.

- Explanation of participant number chosen:
- Many retinal and optic nerve diseases, although varying in etiology, have similar detrimental effects on the photoreceptors, retinal pigment epithelium, or neural tissue. The sample size or number of participants proposed is based on the following:

1. The size of the effect the trial should detect.
2. The Alpha or probability of Type I error (error of reporting the treatment is effective but in reality, it is not).
3. Power or the probability of avoiding Type II error (Beta or the error of reporting the treatment is ineffective but in reality, it is effective).
4. The potential loss of data from inadequate follow-up on the part of the patients over the 5 requested patient exams (1 day, 1 month, 3 months, 6 months, and 12 months).
5. Alpha is set to generally accepted statistical significance for clinical trials, which is $p <$ or equal to 0.05.

With regard to the size of the effect, the trial should detect – we have chosen 0.8 lines of vision (e.g., from 20/200 to 20/100 – or 20/100 to 20/80) or a 10% improvement in visual field for those patients with peripheral vision defects. This is the smallest effect size difference that we believe would have clinical significance.

With Alpha at 0.05 ($p <$ or equal to 0.05) and Beta similarly set to 0.05, the power would be set at 95%. Furthermore, we will assume a standard deviation of 3.3 lines of vision as measured with ETDRS or Snellen Visual Acuity for patients with posterior segment eye disease causing decreased visual acuity between Count Fingers (approximately 20/2000) and 20/40. For 0.8 lines of improvement to occur, the needed number of patients to show, $<$ or equal to 0.05 would be 186, assuming perfect adherence to the follow-up schedule.

"Recent studies show that enrollment rates have decreased from 75% in 2000 to 59% in 2006 and retention rates have fallen from 69% to 48% during same period."

(Getz, "Public Confidence") http://www.ciscrporg/professional/facts_pat.html

If we choose a 60% retention rate, the needed number of patients would be approximately 310.

Therefore, we suggest 500 patients as an appropriate number of participants to be enrolled.

Suggested Reading

Gibson SA, Sanderson HF. Observer variation in ophthalmology. Br J Ophthalmol. 1980;64:457–60.
Knudsen LL. Visual acuity testing in diabetic subjects: the decimal progression chart versus the Freiburg visual acuity test. Graefes Arch Clin Exp Ophthalmol. 2003;241:615–8.

Laidlaw DA, Abbott A, Rosser DA. Development of a clinically feasible logMAR alternative to the Snellen chart: performance of the "compact reduced logMAR" visual acuity chart in amblyopic children. Br J Ophthalmol. 2003;87:1232–4.

Leinonen J, Laakkonen E, Laatikainen L. Random measurement error in visual acuity measurement in clinical settings. Acta Ophthalmol Scand. 2005;83:328–32.

Rosser DA, Laidlaw DA, Murdoch IE. The development of a "reduced logMAR" visual acuity chart for use in routine clinical practice. Br J Ophthalmol. 2001;85:432–6.

Chapter 6
Study Design/Method/Procedures

Summary of Research Design

Preoperative Eye Exam

The preoperative eye exam will include best-corrected visual acuity, external eye exam, intraocular pressures, description of the media and retina, peripheral retinal exam, and examination of the macule and as appropriate testing which may include optical coherence tomography, retinal photography, fluorescein angiography, and visual field testing. All preoperative eye exams will be performed by Dr. Weiss and his staff at his office – -Retina Associates of South Florida located at 5800 Colonial Drive, Suite 300, Margate, Florida 33063 or at 1308 A/B North State Road 7, Margate, FL 33063.

Treatment Location

Treatments will be performed at the Park Creek Surgery Center located at 6806 North State Road 7, Coconut Creek, Florida 33073 at which Dr. Weiss is a member of the medical staff. The procedures will be performed in accordance with all surgery center regulations.

Randomization – no patients are to be randomized. All eligible patients who participate will receive treatment if deemed safe by Dr. Weiss.

© The Author(s), under exclusive license to Springer Nature Switzerland AG 2021
J. N. Weiss, *Retinal and Optic Nerve Stem Cell Surgery*,
https://doi.org/10.1007/978-3-030-60850-7_6

Treatment Procedure

Anesthesia

Anesthesia will be provided by the anesthesia physicians and staff at the Park Creek Surgery Center in accord with good medical judgment and regulations of the surgery center and the State of Florida. This includes all types of anesthesia from local injection to general anesthesia. Typically, the patients have general anesthesia for the bone marrow aspiration and general anesthesia, sedation, or local anesthesia may be used for the injection of the stem cells.

BMSC Collection and Preparation

Approximately 180 cc of bone marrow aspirate will be collected in the operating room, the exact volume being based on medical judgment. The bone marrow aspirate is collected from one or both of the patient's iliac bones in the pelvis and may involve one, two, or more separate sites. The bone marrow aspirate will not leave the operating room. For separation and collection of the mononuclear cell layer including the stem cells and additional components, a medical device called the Angel System, manufactured by Arthrex, Inc or equivalent will be used. The Arthrex Angel System and its components are a Class 2 device per the FDA guidelines.

The collected bone marrow aspirate will be placed in the device, which will separate the components of the bone marrow and isolate the portion containing the adult stem cells. This is done in a completely sterile, automated, and self-contained fashion with minimal manipulation. The device will be operated by Dr. Weiss and/or his assistants under Dr. Weiss's supervision. Approximately 10–15 cc of mononuclear cell material containing the adult stem cells (adult stem cell material) will be available for injection by Dr. Weiss as outlined in the "Eye Treatment" section.

Eye Treatment

Based on the patient's previous examinations/medical evaluation, the stem cell injections will be performed via subtenon and retrobulbar in order to place the stem cells adjacent to one or both eyes. The stem cells may also be provided intraocular, and the delivery method may include intravitreal, intra-optic nerve, intraretinal, subretinal, or retinal vascular injection in one or both eyes.

Dr. Weiss will inject one or both eyes depending on the disease being treated, the vision, and the condition of the eyes. The remaining adult stem cell material may be injected intravenously. Any excess adult stem cell material not used in the course of treatment and any other bone marrow material including other cells and plasma will be discarded in accordance with normal surgery center practice. No material will be retained for future use.

Following treatment, the patient may also receive a steroid injection in one or both eyes treated to reduce inflammation and potentially improve the visual results. This is a commonly performed medication injection following retinal or vitreous surgery.

A subtenon injection is an injection into the space between the tenons tissue surrounding the eye and the sclera or white part of the globe of the eye. The injection is done from the front of the eye and the material allowed to spread under the tenons tissue posteriorly (toward the back of the eye); 1 cc of adult stem cell material may be injected per eye.

A retrobulbar injection is an injection into the posterior orbit (eye socket) and tissues surrounding the eye. From 3 cc of adult stem cell material may be used per eye as determined by Dr. Weiss.

An intravitreal injection is an injection into the vitreous cavity, which is the middle of the ocular globe. The procedure is performed through the sclera or white part of the eye as a direct injection. If this is offered, 0.05 cc will be used per eye as determined by Dr. Weiss.

An intravitreal injection may also be done following vitrectomy on one of the eyes. A vitrectomy is the partial removal of the vitreous of the eye, which is the clear gel inside the middle of the eye. If a vitrectomy is performed, it will only be performed on one eye, and an intravitreal injection of 0.05 cc of adult stem cell material may also be added.

A subretinal injection is the injection beneath the retina between the photoreceptors and the retinal pigment epithelium. This is performed after a vitrectomy is performed. A vitrectomy is the partial removal of the vitreous of the eye, which is the clear gel inside the middle of the eye. After the vitrectomy, a cannula will be inserted beneath the retina and between 0.05 and .1 cc of adult stem cell material will be injected.

An intra-optic nerve injection is an injection just beneath the surface of the optic nerve as the nerve fiber layer enters the optic nerve region or within the parenchyma of the optic nerve itself. The amount injected will be approximately 0.05–0.1 cc of adult stem cell material. This is performed after a vitrectomy.

A retinal vascular injection is an injection into one or more of the retinal blood vessels. The amount injected would be approximately 0.05 cc of adult stem cell material. This would be done after a vitrectomy is performed.

An intraretinal injection is an injection within the retina using a cannula and which includes all the layers of the retina. The amount injected would be approximately 0.05 cc of adult stem cell material. This would be done after a vitrectomy is performed.

Performance of Injections of Adult Stem Cell Material

1. All injections, including subtenon, retrobulbar, intravitreal, intra-optic nerve, intraretinal, subretinal, or retinal vascular injections, are performed while the patient is recumbent. It may also be performed while the patient is seated, if required by their medical condition. Intravenous injection may be performed recumbent or while the patient is sitting.
2. Anesthesia is given as needed for patient comfort and safety under the direction of the anesthesiologist.
3. When the eye is disinfected, the skin around the eye may also be disinfected.
4. The injection occurs under sterile conditions.
5. The adult stem cell material is provided in a syringe under sterile conditions.
6. The adult stem cell material will be provided via subtenon injection into the subtenon space. The injections may be placed in different quadrants (segments) of the eye to best allow the stem cells to spread over the sides and back of the eye.
7. If a retrobulbar injection of the adult stem material is performed, an injection of a small amount of anesthetic may be used prior to a retrobulbar injection.
8. If an intravitreal injection is performed, the material is injected into the center part of the globe.
9. If a subretinal injection is performed, the material is injected beneath the retina. This would be done following vitrectomy, which is the partial or complete removal of the vitreous of the eye using standard intraocular operative approaches for performance of vitrectomy.
10. If an intraretinal injection is performed, the material is injected within the retina. This would be done following vitrectomy, which is the partial or complete removal of the vitreous of the eye using standard intraocular operative approaches for performance of vitrectomy.
11. If an intra-optic nerve injection is performed, the material is injected beneath the surface of the optic nerve or within the parenchyma of the optic nerve. This would be done following vitrectomy, which is the partial or complete removal of the vitreous of the eye using standard intraocular operative approaches for performance of vitrectomy.
12. If a retinal vascular injection is performed, the material is injected within a retinal vessel. This would be done following vitrectomy, which is the partial or complete removal of the vitreous of the eye using standard intraocular operative approaches for performance of vitrectomy.
13. A steroid may be injected in each eye treated if deemed safe.
14. If sufficient adult stem cell material is available, it will be injected intravenously.
15. The patient is then transferred to a bed directly from the treatment table, and wheeled to the recovery room.

Possible Side Effects/Complications

General

This is a surgical procedure involving aspiration of bone marrow and injection of the separated bone marrow stem cell isolate adjacent to the eyes in the orbital area. The procedure will include the administration of medications to provide anesthesia during the procedure. There is always the risk of unanticipated reactions to the procedure itself, the medications, and the anesthesia.

Under very rare circumstances, patients may have serious complications as a result of the procedure or medications including serious abnormal drug reactions, serious allergic reactions, very low blood pressure, seizures, and cardiac or respiratory problems including cardiac or pulmonary arrest. These may result in harm or death.

Bone Marrow Aspiration

Common side effects may include mild local pain, tenderness, and localized bleeding in the area where the physician aspirates the bone marrow. Very rare complications may include infection or bleeding that is difficult to control.

Eye Treatment

With subtenon injections, it is typical to have some mild discomfort or a sense of fullness in the eyes. The eyes may appear red for up to 3–4 weeks. If a retrobulbar injection is given, similar effects can be anticipated.

Exceptionally rare complications, potentially a consequence of subtenon injections, may include infection, local hemorrhage, accidental perforation of the globe, or loss of vision. Perforation is when a needle unintentionally enters the globe itself. Perforation may result in hemorrhage within the eye, injury to the retina, retinal detachment, may require additional surgical procedures to repair, and may result in the loss of vision.

The subtenon injection is done in the front of the eye and visualization is excellent. The risk of accidental perforation of the eye with subtenon injections is reported as less than 0.0008%. In the many thousands of subtenon injections Dr. Weiss has performed, he has not seen these complications.

Subtenon injection of steroids would have a similar extremely small risk of complication such as accidental perforation of the eye. That risk is reported to be less than 0.0008%. Steroids have a small chance of causing glaucoma, which, in most cases, may be treated with topical medications.

Very rare complications potentially a consequence of retrobulbar injection may include infection, retrobulbar hemorrhage, accidental perforation of the globe, damage to the extraocular muscles, damage to the optic nerve, or loss of vision. Retrobulbar injection is also very safe with a less than a 0.014% incidence of perforation reported. In the many thousands of retrobulbar injections Dr. Weiss has performed, he has not seen these complications.

If an intravitreal injection is performed, this may be done in one or both eyes. The injection is done through the sclera or white part of the eye just behind the cornea and iris as a single injection. Intravitreal injections of certain drugs are done commonly for certain retinal diseases including wet macular degeneration, diabetic macular edema and other conditions. Dr. Weiss has done thousands of these drug injections without complication.

The risk of serious complications from any one individual injection is extremely small. There is an extremely small risk of infection inside the eye called endophthalmitis, which can require extensive treatment with antibiotics and/or surgery and may result in loss of vision or of the eye. There is an extremely small risk of damage to the retina or other structures within the eye.

The stem cell material injected is a mixture of cells and may cause a prolonged period of decreased vision, blurriness, cloudiness, or the sense of material floating across the vision. Typically, this clears after a number of weeks as the cells are absorbed; however, it is possible some of these effects may be permanent or require additional surgery to resolve. Intravitreal injections are commonly performed for wet AMD. The incidence of endophthalmitis and retinal complications is less than 4%.

Intravitreal injection may also be performed following a vitrectomy. If this is performed after a vitrectomy the same risks of serious complications as outlined above are seen – however there is additional risk related to the performance of the vitrectomy as outlined below. There is an extremely small risk of infection inside the eye called endophthalmitis, which can require extensive treatment with antibiotics and/or surgery and may result in loss of vision or of the eye. There is a less than 4% risk of developing a retinal detachment, which, in the majority of cases, may be fixed with additional surgery.

There is a small risk of damage to other structures within the eye. The injected stem cell material is a mixture of cells and may cause a prolonged period of decreased vision, blurriness, cloudiness, or the sense of material floating across the vision. Typically, this clears after a number of weeks as the cells are absorbed; however, it is possible that some of these effects may be permanent or require additional surgery to resolve.

If subretinal injection of adult stem cell material is performed, this is done following a vitrectomy. In addition to the possible complications of vitrectomy, specific serious complications of subretinal injection may include retinal detachment, retinal tear, retinal edema or fluid, retinal hemorrhage, choroidal hemorrhage, retinal damage, or damage to other structures within the eye – any of which may cause loss of vision or of the eye. There is an extremely small risk of infection inside the eye called endophthalmitis, which can require extensive treatment with antibiotics and/or surgery and may result in the loss of vision or of the eye.

The injected stem cell material is a mixture of cells and may cause a prolonged period of decreased vision, blurriness, cloudiness, or the sense of material floating across the vision. Typically, this clears after a number of weeks as the cells are absorbed; however, it is possible that some of these effects may be permanent or require additional surgery to resolve. The risk of the above complications of intra-retinal injection is less than 4%.

If an intraretinal injection of adult stem cell material is performed, this is done following a vitrectomy. In addition to the complications of vitrectomy, specific serious complications of subretinal injection may include retinal detachment, retinal tear, retinal edema or fluid, retinal hemorrhage, choroidal hemorrhage, retinal damage, or damage to other structures within the eye – any of which may cause loss of vision or of the eye. There is an extremely small risk of infection inside the eye called endophthalmitis, which can require extensive treatment with antibiotics and/or surgery and may result in loss of vision or of the eye.

The injected stem cell material is a mixture of cells and may cause a prolonged period of decreased vision, blurriness, cloudiness, or the sense of material floating across the vision. Typically, this clears after a number of weeks as the cells are absorbed; however, it is possible some of these effects may be permanent or require additional surgery to resolve. The risk of the above complications of intraretinal injection is less than 4%.

An intra-optic nerve injection of adult stem cell material is performed following a vitrectomy. In addition to the complications of vitrectomy, specific serious complications of intra-optic nerve injection may include retinal detachment, retinal tear, retinal edema or fluid, retinal hemorrhage, choroidal hemorrhage, retinal damage, or damage to other structures within the eye – any of which may cause loss of vision or of the eye. There is an extremely small risk of infection inside the eye called endophthalmitis, which can require extensive treatment with antibiotics and/or surgery and may result in loss of vision or of the eye.

The injected stem cell material is a mixture of cells and may cause a prolonged period of decreased vision, blurriness, cloudiness, or the sense of material floating across the vision. Typically, this clears after a number of weeks as the cells are absorbed; however, it is possible some of these effects may be permanent or may require additional surgery to resolve. The risk of the above complications following intra-optic nerve injection is less than 4%.

A retinal vascular injection of adult stem cell material is performed following a vitrectomy. In addition to the complications of vitrectomy, specific serious complications of retinal vascular injection may include retinal detachment, retinal tear, retinal edema or fluid, retinal hemorrhage, choroidal hemorrhage, retinal damage, or damage to other structures within the eye – any of which may cause loss of vision or of the eye. There is an extremely small risk of infection inside the eye called endophthalmitis, which can require extensive treatment with antibiotics and/or surgery and may result in loss of vision or of the eye.

The injected stem cell material is a mixture of cells and may cause a prolonged period of decreased vision, blurriness, cloudiness, or the sense of material floating across the vision. Typically, this clears after a number of weeks as the cells are absorbed; however, it is possible some of these effects may be permanent or may require additional surgery to resolve. The risk of the above complications is less than 4%.

Vitrectomy is the surgical removal of the clear gel inside the eye called the vitreous. If vitrectomy is performed in order to do a subretinal, intra-optic nerve, intra-retinal, or intravascular injection, there are potential serious complications, which may include retinal detachment, retinal tear, retinal edema or fluid, retinal hemorrhage, choroidal hemorrhage, retinal damage, or damage to other structures within the eye – any of which may cause loss of vision or of the eye. There is an extremely small risk of infection inside the eye called endophthalmitis, which can require extensive treatment with antibiotics and/or surgery and may result in loss of vision or of the eye.

The risk of retinal detachment has been shown to less than 4% from vitrectomy with a 23G instrument. Retinal detachment has a high degree of successful repair. Other complications, such as a retinal tear, have a similarly low incidence and may be addressable with an in-office treatment, such as laser photocoagulation.

Post Procedure Eye Exams

The follow-up eye examinations will be obtained the day after the procedure with Dr. Weiss, and are then requested at 1 month, 3 months, 6 months, and 12 months following the procedure or at the recommended intervals of the eye doctor examining you. Examinations may be performed by Dr. Weiss or by their own eye doctor. Patients agree to allow Dr. Weiss and his associates to release any medical information to their eye doctor and medical doctors. They also agree to provide access to their exams from their eye doctor and medical doctor to Dr. Weiss and his associates.

Collection and Use of Data

Patients give permission for use of their medical information for their own care and for any publication, presentation, or public communication about the procedure and results. In the case of non-direct patient care communication, the patient name and contact information will be held in confidence and not released to protect privacy. However, if required by law, state or federal agencies may be given access to your full name, data, medical records, and information. Access will be granted to the International Cellular Medicine Society Institutional Review Board as they require for monitoring of the IRB.

Analysis of Study Results

Data will be collected and analyzed for significance as outlined under Number 4 – Section F (Number of Participants to be enrolled). Standard statistical methodology will be used.

The purpose of the research is to determine whether bone marrow derived stem cells obtained in the manner outlined and provided to patients in the manner described is an effective treatment for improving visual function by a clinically meaningful amount at the 6-month visit. This will be defined by an improvement of 0.8 lines of vision or a 10% improvement in the area of the visual field. The retinal and optic nerve damage and diseases to be included in the study are those without hope of improvement or are progressive, meaning they normally worsen with time. Many eventually will cause complete blindness. Therefore, improvement to the degree selected will be unprecedented and meaningful.

Monitoring

This will be provided by Dr. Weiss and his staff. Any worsening of vision will be investigated by an eye professional – either a licensed ophthalmologist or optometrist.

Storage of Data

Data will be stored in paper files and will be accessible by Dr. Weiss, his staff, and associates. This will be kept in the usual manner as other medical files and for the required period of time as provided by Florida law.

Confidentiality of Data

All data will be maintained in a confidential manner equal to other medical data and records.

Risk/Benefit Assessment

The risks and discomforts are minimal. Dr. Weiss has performed many thousands of subtenon and retrobulbar injections and the bone marrow aspiration technique is low risk and is performed by a Board-Certified orthopedic surgeon

Risks

General

This is a surgical procedure involving aspiration of bone marrow and injection of the separated bone marrow stem cell isolate adjacent to the eyes in the orbital area. The procedure may include the administration of medications to sedate the patient during the procedure. There is always the risk of unanticipated reactions to the procedure itself or medications. Under very rare circumstances, patients may have serious complications as a result of the procedure or medications including serious abnormal drug reactions, serious allergic reactions, very low blood pressure, and cardiac or respiratory problems including cardiac or pulmonary arrest. These may result in harm to the patient or death.

Bone Marrow Aspiration

Common side effects may include mild local pain, tenderness, and localized bleeding in the area where the doctor aspirates the bone marrow. Very rare complications may include infection or bleeding that is difficult to control.

Eye Treatment

With subtenon injections, it is typical to have some mild discomfort or sense of fullness in the eyes. The eyes may be red for up to 3–4 weeks. If a retrobulbar injection is given, similar effects can be anticipated.

Exceptionally rare complications, potentially a consequence of subtenon injections, may include infection, local hemorrhage, accidental perforation of the globe, or loss of vision. Perforation is when a needle unintentionally enters the globe itself. Perforation may result in hemorrhage within the eye, injury to the retina, retinal detachment, infection, may require additional surgical procedures to repair, and may result in loss of vision.

The subtenon injection is done in the front of the eye and visualization is excellent. The risk of accidental perforation of the eye with subtenon injections is reported as less than 0.0008%. In the many thousands of subtenon injections Dr. Weiss has performed, he has not seen these complications.

Very rare complications, potentially a consequence of retrobulbar injection, may include infection, retrobulbar hemorrhage, accidental perforation of the globe, damage to extraocular muscles, damage to optic nerve, or loss of vision. Retrobulbar injection is also very safe with a less than a 0.014% incidence of perforation reported. In the many thousands of retrobulbar injections Dr. Weiss has performed, he has not seen these complications.

Similarly, complications from intravitreal injections are extremely rare. Many hundreds of thousands of intravitreal drug injections are done every year in the United States primarily for wet macular degeneration (AMD) and diabetic retinopathy. The safety profile is extremely favorable.

The risk of other intraocular injections including intraretinal, subretinal, intraoptic nerve, and retinal vasculature injections is estimated to be less that less than 4% per injection.

The risk of vitrectomy as performed by Dr. Weiss is favorable with a retinal detachment risk of less than 4%. Retinal detachment is a complication, which has a very high probability of successful repair. Given the blinding nature of many of the diseases causing retinal and optic nerve damage and the poor vision many patients will have treated, the risk/benefit ratio is very favorable.

Prevention of Risks

Medical clearance is required for all patients treated. Typically, for surgical procedures any anticoagulants are discontinued 7–10 days prior to a procedure if the primary care physician believes this to be safe for the patient.

Dr. Weiss has the experience to minimize any risk to the patient for all ophthalmic procedures. Dr. Silberfarb, the orthopedic surgeon, similarly has extensive experience and will perform the technique in a way to minimize risks.

Procedures will be done in one of the assigned operating rooms of the Park Creek Surgical Center. Standard procedures and staffing as required by Florida law for surgical procedures will be provided, which may include a surgical technician(s) or scrub nurse(s). Anesthesia services will be provided by one of their Board-Certified anesthesiologists and their staff. Equipment will include all supportive equipment required for safe operative care of patients and required by Florida law and certification organizations. This will include anesthetic and pharmacologic drugs and equipment for routine operative patient care and anesthesia administration as well as that needed for emergent care (respiratory or cardiac support).

Adverse Events

Any Adverse Events (AE) or Serious Adverse Events (SAE) will be managed by the physicians caring for the patient at the time of the event. An Adverse Event will be defined as an event related to the procedure that has a high risk to cause permanent loss of vision or health to the patient.

An Adverse Event will be reported to ICMS IRB within 60 days of documentation. These may include anesthesia events, retinal detachment, endophthalmitis, or osteomyelitis requiring treatment. A Serious Adverse Event will be defined as permanent loss of vision or permanent medical injury to the patient as a result of the procedure and will be reported to ICMS IRB within 45 business days of their documentation.

Benefits

Dr. Weiss has personally observed improvement in visual function including visual fields and visual acuity in patients he has treated in the United States, Europe, and Dubai. We also have anecdotal reports of other patient improvements.

Participant Recruitment and Informed Consent

Recruiting

Recruiting will be brought to the attention of potential patients through announcements on the Internet, email, press releases, direct communications with healthcare providers, and potentially paid advertising in accordance with normal and ethical recruiting practices. Recruiting will continue until 500 patients have been enrolled. No coercion will be used. In the course of providing information about the study, it will be communicated that patients will be participating in a clinical study conducted under an IRB protocol approved and monitored by the International Cellular Medicine Society.

Length of Study

The study will begin on the date of IRB approval and continue until one (1) year following the treatment of the last recruited patient.

Informed Consent/Assent

See Informed Consent Below

Chapter 7
Informed Consent

Informed Consent and Permission

Bone Marrow Derived Stem Cell Ophthalmology Treatment Study II

- Jeffrey N. Weiss, MD
- Retina Associates of South Florida
- 5800 Colonial Drive, Suite 300
- Margate, Florida 33063
- Telephone 954–975-0044

Introduction

To decide whether or not you want to have the Bone Marrow Derived Stem Cell Ophthalmology Treatment (called "the procedure" in this document) – also known as an Adult Stem Cell Treatment, the risks and possible benefits are described in this form so that you can make an informed decision. This process is known as informed consent. This consent form describes the purpose, procedures, possible benefits, and risks of the procedure. You may have a copy of this form to review at your leisure or to ask advice from others.

Dr. Weiss and his associates will answer any questions you may have about this form or about the procedure. Please read this document carefully and do not hesitate to ask anything about this information. This form may contain words that you do not understand. Please ask Dr. Weiss or his associates to explain the words or information that you do not understand. After reading (or having it read to you) the consent form, if you would like to be treated you will be asked to sign this form.

© The Author(s), under exclusive license to Springer Nature Switzerland AG 2021   49
J. N. Weiss, *Retinal and Optic Nerve Stem Cell Surgery*,
https://doi.org/10.1007/978-3-030-60850-7_7

Background

Bone marrow derived stem cells (BMSC) are adult stem cells that come from a patient's own bone marrow. There is anecdotal evidence that patients with certain eye diseases have improved visual function following treatment with BMSC. The exact mechanisms by which adult stem cells can provide improvement is complex and still undergoing assessment in the medical and scientific community. Adult stem cell treatments have been performed and continue to be performed in various parts of the world including the United States for a number of medical conditions. It is unknown whether this treatment will be of benefit in your particular eye disease.

Terms of the Study

Dr. Weiss will determine if you and your eye condition are eligible for inclusion in the study. If you have been approved for inclusion in the study you are being asked to participate in a clinical research study to determine if the use of bone marrow derived stem cell (BMSC) injections can benefit damaged retinal and optic nerve tissue and improve visual function for patients. While there have been many patients worldwide treated with BMSC in various ways including treatment for retinal and optic nerve disease, sufficient proof such as may be demonstrated with scientific studies, has not been developed to convince the majority of physicians the procedure is of benefit. The purpose of this study is to determine if improvement in visual function–central visual acuity and/or peripheral vision can be obtained by using BMSC injections.

The type of injection used will be determined by Dr. Weiss after your eye examination. The injections may include retrobulbar (behind the eye), subtenon (underneath the layer just outside the eye called the tenons layer), intravitreal (within the vitreous cavity or vitreous, which is the clear gel in the middle of the eye), subretinal (beneath the retina), intra-optic nerve (within the optic nerve), intraretinal (within the retina), retinal vascular (into a retinal vessel), and intravenous (into the vein and blood circulation).

If subretinal, intra-optic nerve, intraretinal, or retinal vascular is offered, the eye will need to undergo a surgical operation called a vitrectomy. A vitrectomy may also be suggested prior to an intravitreal injection in one eye. You understand that participation in this study is voluntary and the treatment of your illness is not dependent upon you participating in this study.

You may be offered subthreshold laser (not visible to the surgeon) or visible laser photocoagulation of the retina. This is the use of laser photocoagulation to create one or more areas of either not visible or visible damage to the retina that may attract and hold the stem cells.

There will be 500 participants enrolled in the study at one site in the United States. It is anticipated you will participate in this research study for 1 year.

Reproductive Information for Females

There is no evidence treatment with autologous bone marrow derived stem cells have adverse effects on human reproduction or a developing unborn fetus. However, female patients who are pregnant or attempting to become pregnant should not undergo treatment. It is suggested that female patients do not attempt to become pregnant for at least 3 months following treatment. If female, in signing this informed consent you attest that you believe that you are not pregnant and if you are of childbearing potential, you are using an adequate form of birth control and will continue to do so for 3 months following treatment.

Benefits/Outcome of Treatment

The potential benefits of this treatment may include improvement in visual function. Visual function includes visual acuity, which is a measurement of the ability to see clearly at distance or near. It also includes peripheral vision, which is the ability to see to the side of the central vision. However, it is possible your visual function may experience no change or worsen. Any improvement may take several months. At this time, Dr. Weiss cannot make predictions as to the effectiveness of the stem cell treatment for individual patients.

In signing this informed consent, you acknowledge that no promise of beneficial results has been made to you, nor have any guarantees been offered, either formally or implied, that treatment with bone marrow derived stem cells will be successful or of benefit.

Description of Procedure

In this procedure, the bone marrow derived stem cells (BMSC) will be isolated from your bone marrow and then the stem cell material obtained will be injected in the subtenon space, in the retrobulbar space, in the intravitreal space, and the subretinal space depending on Dr. Weiss's assessment of your vision and ocular condition. Both eyes will be treated if this is believed safe and beneficial by Dr. Weiss. If there is sufficient stem cell material obtained, the remaining isolate will also be reinjected intravenously.

This procedure is considered invasive and includes removing bone marrow from the iliac crest (one or both) of your pelvis and the injection of the separated stem cells adjacent to in your eye(s). The removal of bone marrow from a patient's pelvis is an established medical procedure. However, the use of bone marrow derived stem cells in ophthalmology is not considered to be evidence-based medicine. This means that there is not enough scientific evidence to determine if this procedure is beneficial to the visual function of patients.

Follow-Up Exams

The first follow-up eye exam must be obtained on the day after treatment with Dr. Weiss at his office. If you are in Arm 3, Dr. Weiss will likely require you to have a follow-up at 10–14 days following the procedure – which may be done with Dr. Weiss or your own ophthalmologist. It is then strongly suggested that the patient have follow-up exams at 1 month, 3 months, 6 months, and 12 months following the procedure with either Dr. Weiss or their own licensed ophthalmologist or optometrist. The follow-up exams are extremely important to monitor the health of your eyes.

If you notice any sudden changes or deterioration in the eyes or vision following the procedure such as pain, decreased vision, redness, discharge, cloudy appearance to the cornea, floaters, or any other development that is different from your normal experience, please get in touch with Dr. Weiss or your local eye care provider immediately as this could represent a threat to your vision or health.

This permission also provides for access to your follow-up eye exams to Dr. Weiss and his associates and the ability to discuss your treatment and results freely with your health providers. We strongly request all follow-up exams be forwarded to Dr. Weiss and his associates. This may require that the patient giving permission to their eye care doctor to forward their records or may involve the patient obtaining those records and then forwarding them to Dr. Weiss.

Alternative Treatments

Some of the eye diseases that are offered BMSC treatment may have existing drug, laser photocoagulation, or surgical treatments that have scientific evidence or general medical community acceptance for use in maintaining or improving visual function. If there are such existing treatments, Dr. Weiss will inform you and you will have the choice as to whether or not to have this stem cell procedure.

If you elect to undergo stem cell treatment, it is recommended that you continue all current medical therapies prescribed by your existing eye care doctor including their recommended follow-up exams until they can examine you and make their own assessment of the need for their therapies or examinations. In signing this informed consent, you acknowledge you are aware of potential alternative treatments as indicated by Dr. Weiss and elect to undergo the stem cell procedure.

Potential Alternative Treatments Identified by Dr. Weiss

_____

_____

Medical Treatments and Costs

This procedure is not considered evidence based by insurance companies. You understand that your participation in this study is at your own expense and will not be reimbursed by any insurance company.

Should a study-related medical problem or injury occur, appropriate medical care, as determined by your physician or ophthalmologist, may be provided by your physician, Dr. Weiss, or your own ophthalmologist.

You understand you will be financially responsible for such medical treatment although your insurance company may cover any such treatment under your existing policy. You understand that no additional financial compensation will be available for any injury resulting from your participation. This does not constitute a waiver of any rights that you may have under Federal or State laws and regulations.

Preoperative Eye Exam

The preoperative eye exam will include best-corrected visual acuity, external eye exam, intraocular pressures, description of the media and retina, peripheral retinal exam, and examination of the macule and as appropriate testing which may include optical coherence tomography, retinal photography, fluorescein angiography, and visual field testing. All preoperative eye exams will be performed by Dr. Weiss and his staff at his office – Retina Associates of South Florida located at 5800 Colonial Drive, Suite 300, Margate, Florida 33063.

Treatment Location

Treatments will be performed at the Park Creek Surgery Center located at 6806 North State Road 7, Coconut Creek, Florida 33073, at which Dr. Weiss is a member of the medical staff. The procedures will be performed in accordance with all surgery center regulations.

Acceptance of Risks

The treatment provided is experimental and no guarantees are provided as to the outcome of the procedure. The vision may become better, stay the same, or worsen. I accept these risks freely and agree to hold harmless Dr. Weiss and Retina Associates of South Florida; Dr. Levy and MD Stem Cells; and the personnel who participate in performing the procedure.

Initial_____

Medical Clearance

Medical clearance for anesthesia and surgery will be obtained by the patient through their own medical doctor prior to the procedure and provided to Dr. Weiss and the associated physicians and staff of the Park Creek Surgery Center. The medical clearance must give permission for the use of general anesthesia and provide such laboratory tests and examination as Dr. Weiss and the additional physicians at Park Creek Surgery Center believe are needed to properly assess your risks and provide proper care for you while you undergo the procedure.

Anesthesia

Anesthesia will be provided by the anesthesia physicians and staff at the Park Creek Surgery Center in accordance with good medical judgment and regulations of the surgery center and the State of Florida. This includes all types of anesthesia from local injection to general anesthesia. Typically, the patients have general anesthesia for the bone marrow aspiration and general anesthesia, sedation, or local anesthesia may be used for the injection of the stem cells.

Treatment Procedure

Approximately 180 cc of bone marrow aspirate will be collected in the operating room by Dr. Steven Silberfarb, a Florida licensed orthopedic surgeon and staff member of the Park Creek Surgery Center, the exact volume being based on his medical judgment. The bone marrow aspirate is collected from one or both of the patient's iliac bones in the pelvis and may involve one, two, or more separate sites. The bone marrow aspirate will not leave the operating room.

For separation and collection of the mononuclear cell layer including the stem cells, a medical device called the Arthrex Angel system will be used. The collected bone marrow aspirate will be placed in the device, which will separate the components of the bone marrow and isolate the portion containing the adult stem cells. This is done in a completely sterile, automated, and self-contained fashion with minimal manipulation. The device will be operated by Dr. Weiss and/or his assistants under Dr. Weiss's supervision. Approximately 8 cc of mononuclear cell material containing the adult stem cells (adult stem cell material) will be available for ocular injection by Dr. Weiss as outlined in the "Eye Treatment" section.

Eye Treatment

Based on the patient's previous examinations/medical evaluation, the stem cell injections will be performed via subtenon and retrobulbar in order to place the stem cells adjacent to one or both eyes. The stem cells may also be provided as an intra-vitreal, intra-optic nerve, intraretinal, subretinal, or retinal vascular injection in one or both eyes. Dr. Weiss will inject one or both eyes depending on the disease being treated, the vision, and the condition of the eyes.

The remaining adult stem cell material may be injected intravenously. Any excess adult stem cell material not used in the course of treatment and any other bone mar-row material including other cells and plasma will be discarded in accordance with normal surgery center practice. No material will be retained for future use.

Following treatment, the patient may also receive an injection of steroids in the eyes treated to reduce inflammation and potentially improve the visual results. This is a commonly performed medication injection following retinal or vitreous surgery.

A subtenon injection is an injection into the space between the tenons tissue sur-rounding the eye and the sclera or white part of the globe of the eye. The injection is done from the front of the eye and the material allowed to spread under the tenons tissue posteriorly (toward the back of the eye); 1 cc of adult stem cell material may be injected per eye.

A retrobulbar injection is an injection into the posterior orbit (eye socket) and tissues surrounding the eye; 3 cc of adult stem cell material may be used per eye as determined by Dr. Weiss.

An intravitreal injection is an injection into the vitreous cavity, which is the mid-dle of the ocular globe. If this is done as a simple procedure, it is done through the sclera or white part of the eye as a direct injection. If this is offered, 0.05 cc will be used per eye as determined by Dr. Weiss.

An intravitreal injection may also be done following vitrectomy on one of the eyes. A vitrectomy is the partial removal of the vitreous of the eye, which is the clear gel inside the middle of the eye. If a vitrectomy is performed, it will only be per-formed on one eye, and the volume injected will be from 0.05 to 0.1 cc of adult stem cell material.

A subretinal injection is the injection beneath the retina between the photorecep-tors and the retinal pigment epithelium. This is performed after a vitrectomy is performed. A vitrectomy is the partial removal of the vitreous of the eye, which is the clear gel inside the middle of the eye. After the vitrectomy, a cannula will be inserted beneath the retina and between 0.05 and 0.1 cc of adult stem cell material will be injected.

An intra-optic nerve injection is an injection just beneath the surface of the optic nerve as the nerve fiber layer enters the optic nerve region or within the parenchyma of the optic nerve itself. The amount injected will be approximately 0.05 cc of adult stem cell material. This is performed after a vitrectomy is performed.

A retinal vascular injection is an injection into one or more of the retinal blood vessels. The amount injected would be approximately 0.05 cc of adult stem cell material. This would be done after a vitrectomy is performed.

An intraretinal injection is an injection within the retina using a cannula and which includes all the layers of the retina. The amount injected would be approximately 0.05 cc of adult stem cell material. This would be done after a vitrectomy is performed.

Performance of Injections of Adult Stem Cell Material

1. The subtenon and/or retrobulbar and/or intravitreal injections and/or subretinal injections are performed while the patient is recumbent. It may be performed while the patient is seated if required by their medical condition.
2. Anesthesia is given as needed for patient comfort and safety under the direction of the anesthesiologist.
3. When the eye is disinfected, the skin around the eye may also be disinfected.
4. The injection occurs under sterile conditions.
5. The adult stem cell material is provided in a syringe under sterile conditions.
6. The adult stem cell material will be provided via subtenon injection into the subtenon space. The injections may be placed in different quadrants (segments) of the eye to best allow the stem cells to spread over the sides and back of the eye.
7. If a retrobulbar injection of the adult stem material is performed, and the patient is not under anesthesia, an injection of a small amount of anesthetic may be used prior to a retrobulbar injection.
8. If an intravitreal injection is performed, the material is injected into the center part of the globe.
9. If a subretinal injection is performed, the material is injected beneath the retina. This would be done following vitrectomy, which is the partial or complete removal of the vitreous of the eye using standard intraocular operative approaches for the performance of a vitrectomy.
10. If an intraretinal injection is performed the material is injected within the retina. This would be done following a vitrectomy, which is the partial or complete removal of the vitreous of the eye using standard intraocular operative approaches for the performance of vitrectomy.
11. If an intra-optic nerve injection is performed, the material is injected beneath the surface of the optic nerve or within the parenchyma of the optic nerve. This

would be done following the vitrectomy, which is the partial or complete removal of the vitreous of the eye using standard intraocular operative approaches for performance of vitrectomy.

12. If a retinal vascular injection is performed, the material is injected within a retinal vessel. This would be done following the vitrectomy, which is the partial or complete removal of the vitreous of the eye using standard intraocular operative approaches for performance of vitrectomy.

13. A steroid will be injected in each eye treated if deemed safe.

14. If sufficient adult stem cell material is available, it may be injected intravenously.

15. The patient is then transferred to a bed directly from the treatment table, and wheeled to the recovery room.

Possible Side Effects/Complications

Please feel free to discuss any of these potential side effects or complications with Dr. Weiss or the other physicians involved in your care.

General

This is a surgical procedure involving the aspiration of bone marrow and injection of the separated bone marrow stem cell isolate adjacent to your eyes in the orbital area. The procedure will include the administration of medications to provide anesthesia during the procedure. There is always the risk of unanticipated reactions to the procedure itself, the medications, and the anesthesia. Under very rare circumstances, patients may have serious complications as a result of the procedure or medications including serious abnormal drug reactions, serious allergic reactions, very low blood pressure, seizures, and cardiac or respiratory problems including cardiac or pulmonary arrest. These may result in harm to your body or death.

Bone Marrow Aspiration

Common side effects may include mild local pain, tenderness, and localized bleeding in the area where the doctor aspirates the bone marrow. Very rare complications may include infection or bleeding that is difficult to control.

Eye Treatment

With subtenon injections, it is typical to have some mild discomfort or sense of fullness in the eyes. The eyes may appear red for up to 2–3 weeks. If a retrobulbar
injection is given, similar effects can be anticipated.

Exceptionally rare complications, potentially a consequence of subtenon injections, may include infection, local hemorrhage, accidental perforation of the globe,
or loss of vision. Perforation is when a needle unintentionally enters the globe itself.
Perforation may result in hemorrhage within the eye, injury to the retina, retinal
detachment, may require additional surgical procedures to repair, and may result in
the loss of vision.

The subtenon injection is done in the front of the eye and visualization is excellent. The risk of accidental perforation of the eye with a subtenon injection is
reported as less than 0.0008%. In the many thousands of subtenon injections Dr.
Weiss has performed, he has not seen these complications.

Very rare complications, potentially a consequence of retrobulbar injection may
include infection, retrobulbar hemorrhage, accidental perforation of the globe, damage to extraocular muscles, damage to optic nerve, or loss of vision. Retrobulbar
injection is also very safe with a less than a 0.014% incidence of perforation
reported. In the many thousands of retrobulbar injections Dr. Weiss has performed,
he has not seen these complications.

If an intravitreal injection is performed, this may be done in one or both eyes.
The injection is done through the sclera or white part of the eye just behind the cornea and iris as a single injection. Intravitreal injections of certain drugs are done
commonly for certain retinal diseases including wet macular degeneration, diabetic
macular edema, and other conditions. Dr. Weiss has done thousands of these drug
injections without complication.

The risk of serious complications from any one individual injection is extremely
small. There is an extremely small risk of infection inside the eye called endophthalmitis, which can require extensive treatment with antibiotics and/or surgery and
may result in the loss of vision or of the eye. There is a small risk of damage to the
retina or other structures within the eye.

The stem cell material injected is a mixture of cells and may cause a prolonged
period of decreased vision, blurriness, cloudiness, or the sense of material floating
across the vision. Typically, this clears after 1–3 months as the cells are absorbed.
However, it is possible some of these effects may be permanent or require additional
surgery to resolve.

An intravitreal injection may also be performed following a vitrectomy. If this is
performed after a vitrectomy, the same risks of serious complications as outlined
above are seen; however, there is additional risk related to the performance of the
vitrectomy as outlined below. There is an extremely small risk of infection inside
the eye called endophthalmitis, which can require extensive treatment with antibiotics and/or surgery and may result in loss of vision or of the eye.

There is an extremely small risk of damage to the retina or other structures within the eye. The stem cell material injected is a mixture of cells and may cause a prolonged period of decreased vision, blurriness, cloudiness, or the sense of material floating across the vision. Typically, this clears after a number of weeks as the cells are absorbed; however, it is possible some of these effects may be permanent or require additional surgery to resolve.

The subretinal injection of adult stem cell material is performed following a vitrectomy. In addition to the complications of vitrectomy, specific serious complications of subretinal injection may include retinal detachment, retinal tear, retinal edema or fluid, retinal hemorrhage, choroidal hemorrhage, retinal damage, or damage to other structures within the eye – any of which may cause loss of vision or of the eye.

There is an extremely small risk of infection inside the eye called endophthalmitis, which can require extensive treatment with antibiotics and/or surgery and may result in loss of vision or of the eye. The stem cell material injected is a mixture of cells and may cause a prolonged period of decreased vision, blurriness, cloudiness, or the sense of material floating across the vision. Typically, this clears after 1–3 months as the cells are absorbed; however, it is possible some of these effects may be permanent or require additional surgery to resolve. It is estimated that the above complications of subretinal injection would be less than 4%.

If intraretinal injection of adult stem cell material is performed, this is done following a vitrectomy. In addition to the complications of vitrectomy as outlined below, specific serious complications of subretinal injection may include retinal detachment, retinal tear, retinal edema or fluid, retinal hemorrhage, choroidal hemorrhage, retinal damage, or damage to other structures within the eye – any of which may cause loss of vision or of the eye. There is an extremely small risk of infection inside the eye called endophthalmitis, which can require extensive treatment with antibiotics and/or surgery and may result in loss of vision or of the eye.

The stem cell material injected is a mixture of cells and may cause a prolonged period of decreased vision, blurriness, cloudiness, or the sense of material floating across the vision. Typically, this clears after a number of weeks as the cells are absorbed; however, it is possible some of these effects may be permanent or require additional surgery to resolve. The risk of the above complications of intraretinal injection is less than 4%.

If an intra-optic nerve injection of adult stem cell material is performed, this is done following a vitrectomy. In addition to the complications of vitrectomy, specific serious complications of intra-optic nerve injection may include retinal detachment, retinal tear, retinal edema or fluid, retinal hemorrhage, choroidal hemorrhage, retinal damage, or damage to other structures within the eye – any of which may cause loss of vision or of the eye. There is an extremely small risk of infection inside the eye called endophthalmitis, which can require extensive treatment with antibiotics and/or surgery and may result in the loss of vision or of the eye.

The stem cell material injected is a mixture of cells and may cause a prolonged period of decreased vision, blurriness, cloudiness, or the sense of material floating across the vision. Typically, this clears after a number of weeks as the cells are absorbed; however, it is possible some of these effects may be permanent or require additional surgery to resolve. The risk of the above complications following intra-optic nerve injection is less than 4%.

A retinal vascular injection of adult stem cell material is performed following a vitrectomy. In addition to the complications of vitrectomy, specific serious complications of retinal vascular injection may include retinal detachment, retinal tear, retinal edema or fluid, retinal hemorrhage, choroidal hemorrhage, retinal damage, or damage to other structures within the eye – any of which may cause loss of vision or of the eye. There is an extremely small risk of infection inside the eye called endophthalmitis, which may require extensive treatment with antibiotics and/or surgery and may result in loss of vision or of the eye.

The stem cell material injected is a mixture of cells and may cause a prolonged period of decreased vision, blurriness, cloudiness, or the sense of material floating across the vision. Typically, this clears after a number of weeks as the cells are absorbed; however, it is possible that some of these effects may be permanent or require additional surgery to resolve. The risk of the above complications is less than 4%.

If you are offered subthreshold laser (not visible to the surgeon) or visible laser photocoagulation of the retina, this is the use of laser photocoagulation to create one or more areas of either not visible or visible damage to the retina that may attract and hold the stem cells. The risk of subthreshold laser or visible laser photocoagulation is inadvertent damage to the vision.

Vitrectomy is the surgical removal of the clear gel inside the eye. If vitrectomy is performed in order to do a subretinal injection or an intravitreal injection, there are potential serious complications, which may include retinal detachment, retinal tear, retinal edema or fluid, retinal hemorrhage, choroidal hemorrhage, retinal damage, or damage to other structures within the eye – any of which may cause loss of vision or of the eye. There is an extremely small risk of infection inside the eye called endophthalmitis, which can require extensive treatment with antibiotics and/or surgery and may result in loss of vision or of the eye.

The risk of retinal detachment following vitrectomy is less than 4%. Retinal detachment has a high degree of successful repair. Other complications have a similarly very low incidence and may be addressable with in office treatment such as laser photocoagulation. Dr. Weiss will only perform vitrectomy on those patients he believes offer a very low risk of complications.

- Retina. 2011 May;31(5):902–8. https://doi.org/10.1097/IAE.0b013e3182069aa4.
- Does 23-gauge sutureless vitrectomy modify the risk of postoperative retinal detachment after macular surgery? A comparison with 20-gauge vitrectomy. Le Rouic JF, Becquet F, Ducournau D.

Post Procedure Eye Exams

The follow-up eye exams will be obtained the day after the procedure with Dr. Weiss, and are then requested at 1 month, 3 months, 6 months, and 12 months following the procedure or at the recommended intervals of the eye doctor examining you. Examinations may be performed by Dr. Weiss or by their own eye doctor. Patients agree to allow Dr. Weiss and his associates to release any medical information to their eye doctor and medical doctors. They also agree to provide access to their examinations from their eye doctor and medical doctor to Dr. Weiss and his associates.

Collection and Use of Data

Patients give permission for the use of their medical information for their own care and for any publication, presentation, or public communication about the procedure and results. In the case of non-direct patient care communication, the patient name and contact information will be held in confidence and not released to protect your privacy. However, if required by law, state or federal agencies may be given access to your full name, data, medical records, and information.

Confidentiality of Records

You understand that your identity and certain information pertaining to you that is collected for this study will remain confidential. However, in order to meet the obligations of Federal law, you understand that records from this study may be subject to review by representatives of the International Cellular Medicine Society Institutional Review Board and authorized Food and Drug Administration or other government regulatory age personnel. You hereby consent to such review and disclosure.

Available Information

You understand that any significant new information developed during the course of this study, which may relate to your willingness to continue as a participant, will be provided to you.

If you have any questions or desire further information with respect to this study, or if you experience a study-related injury, you should contact:

Jeffrey N. Weiss, MD   Steven Levy, MD
Principal Investigator   Study Director
5800 Colonial Drive, Suite 300   412 Main Street, Suite I
Margate, FL 33063.   Ridgefield, CT 06877
Phone: (954) 975-0044   Phone: (203) 423-9494

If you wish to contact an impartial third party not associated with this study, you may contact:

Reed Davis at 702-664-0017.

Termination

You understand that your participation in this study is voluntary and you are under no obligation to participate. Your decision on whether to participate in the study will in no way impact upon the treatment you will receive. You may refuse to participate or leave the study at any time without penalty or loss of benefits to which you are otherwise entitled. If you choose not to participate, or to discontinue your participation in this study, Jeffrey N. Weiss, M.D., and his associates will continue to take care of your illness to the best of their ability.

In addition, you understand that your participation may be terminated by Jeffrey N. Weiss, M.D., and/or your physician without regard to your consent, should he/she determine that continued participation would be detrimental to you in any way. You understand that at the completion of the study, you may not be able to continue participation.

Participant Statement and Authorization

In affixing my signature, I acknowledge I have read or had read to me this informed consent and permission form, that all my questions have been answered and that I fully understand the information it contains. I consent to the procedure of Bone Marrow Stem Cell treatment for my eye disease as performed by Dr. Jeffrey Weiss and his associates. This informed consent and permission (also called an authorization) will have no end date

_____

Printed Name of Patient

_____   _____

Signature of Patient   Date

_____

Name of and Relationship of Responsible Party if patient unable to sign

_____   _____

Signature of Responsible Party if patient unable to sign   Date

_____

Printed Name of Person Explaining Consent

_____   _____

Signature of Person Explaining Consent   Date

Chapter 8
Procedure: Additional Patient Explanation

Patients first contact the SCOTS Study Director, Dr. Steven Levy, the President of MD Stem Cells. Dr. Levy provides information and manages the logistics and data for the study. Patient ophthalmic records are sent to Dr. Levy at stevenlevy@mdstemcells.com.

Dr. Levy forwards the records to Dr. Jeffrey Weiss, the Principal Investigator of SCOTS and a practicing retinal specialist in Margate, Florida, for review. Dr. Weiss independently determines patient eligibility. He will also select the best procedure for the patient. Dr. Weiss performs all ophthalmic surgeries.

The surgery is usually performed using monitored or general anesthesia, and takes less than 1 hour. A state-of-the-art fully licensed outpatient surgery center is used for all procedures. An orthopedic surgeon performs the bone marrow aspiration and the bone marrow fraction (BMF), which consists of the stem cells and multiple growth factors, is isolated using our protocol in an FDA-approved Class 2 device.

In SCOTS, there is the choice of three ophthalmic procedures:

- Arm 1 consists of a retrobulbar and a subtenon injection of the BMF. A retrobulbar injection is the placement of cells behind the eye. A subtenon injection is the placement of cells between the sclera, or white part of the eye, and the overlying transparent tissue.
- Arm 2 consists of the Arm 1 procedures and an intravitreal injection. An intravitreal injection is injecting the cells into the eye.
- Arm 3 is a vitrectomy and a subtenon injection. A vitrectomy is a surgical procedure that is used to remove the clear vitreous body gel from inside the eye. The vitreous material is replaced with a saline solution. The vitrectomy allows the surgeon access to directly inject cells into the optic nerve or under the retina.

© The Author(s), under exclusive license to Springer Nature Switzerland AG 2021
J. N. Weiss, *Retinal and Optic Nerve Stem Cell Surgery*,
https://doi.org/10.1007/978-3-030-60850-7_8

The procedures are tailored for the individual patient. The patient may have Arm 1 or 2 in one or both eyes, but Arm 3 is reserved for one eye, and for the eye with the worse visual acuity. As of this date, we have performed the SCOTS surgery on more than 500 patients, and more than 900 eyes.

Experience has shown that the direct placement of the BMF under the retina may be beneficial for certain diseases that affect the macula – the center portion of the retina. However, for many retinal diseases including different macular diseases, improvements in vision have been seen in patients receiving Arm 1 or 2 injections alone.

Similarly, direct injection of the optic nerve may be provided in specific cases as the cells seem to remain over time. However, the optic nerve actually forms from the nerve fiber layer, a portion of the retina – therefore Arm 1 or 2 injections alone are sufficient to see improvements in many cases.

There have been no complications in patients undergoing Arm 1 or 2. In the first 100 Arm 3 cases, there were three retinal detachments where a commercially available needle was used to inject the cells. All three cases were successfully repaired. As a result of this experience, Dr. Weiss developed his own subretinal needles and since utilizing these needles, there have been no retinal detachments.

Experience has shown that eyes in each of the categories improve. The choice of which Arm of the procedure the patient receives is based on the ophthalmic history and the clinical examination.

In Arm 3 for retinal cases, Dr. Weiss performs a vitrectomy and then using a needle of his design, places the BMF in the area of atrophic retina.

In the Arm 3 optic nerve cases, following the vitrectomy, there is a direct injection of the BMF cells into the optic nerve. If the visual acuity is sufficient to perform a visual field test, Dr. Weiss uses the field to guide the injection into atrophic nerve.

In either Arm 1 or 2, the eye is not patched. The eye undergoing Arm 3 is patched for 24 hours.

The patients are instructed to not rub their eyes, to avoid heavy lifting and straining, and in the Arm 2 and 3 eyes, to keep their "head above their heart" and sleep on two pillows until the "floaters" are gone.

It is important to note that the BMF is red in color. Our cell separation protocol has been developed over 5 years and been modified and improved multiple times in order to minimize the presence of red blood cells.

Typically Arm 1 and Arm 2 patients will postoperatively exhibit inferior orbital discoloration and subconjunctival redness. This is the color of the BMF, it is not hemorrhage. Arm 2 patients will look like there is a "vitreous hemorrhage," it is not hemorrhage, but the BMF.

The intravitreal BMF generally is clumped inferiorly, but in a vitrectomized eye, or an eye that has experienced a posterior vitreous detachment with a very "liquid" vitreous, the cells will dissipate giving the impression of a vitreous hemorrhage. This may also be seen in Arm 3 eyes treated for a retinal condition in that some of the BMF may remain in the vitreous cavity. In those Arm 3 eyes that underwent direct injection of the BMF into the optic disc, though there may not be any BMF in the vitreous cavity at the conclusion of surgery, some of the BMF material may be visible overlying the optic disc on the first postoperative day.

Knowing what to expect is important. We have had one case in which the patient returned home after SCOTS treatment, her ophthalmologist saw a "vitreous hemorrhage" and he immediately performed a vitrectomy to remove the BMF that we placed!

Arm 1 and Arm 2 patients report that their eyes feel "scratchy." The discomfort is generally gone by the first postoperative day. Arm 3 eyes are patched until the first postoperative day, and then the patient may feel a foreign body sensation for a few days. All patients report either slight or no hip discomfort after surgery. For postoperative pain only, Acetaminophen 500 mg is recommended as needed. Nonsteroidal anti-inflammatories are not recommended during the postoperative period as they may promote hemorrhaging.

The patients are instructed to refrain from straining activities, such as heavy lifting and to keep their head "above their heart" for 1 month after surgery. The Arm 3 patients are advised to wear glasses or a metal shield when they sleep, for 1 month after surgery.

Data are collected at 1, 3, 6, and 12 months postoperatively. The post-surgical examinations are generally performed by the patient's local eye doctor. The information we request is visual acuity, eye pressure, anterior and posterior segment examinations, fundus photography, optical coherence tomography (OCT), and visual fields.

The periorbital and subconjunctival redness and the intravitreal BMF material generally resolve with 1 month. We have seen improvements in visual acuity or visual field on the first postoperative day in approximately 10% of cases, although improvements are generally noted from 4 to 6 months after the procedure. We have had one patient who suddenly experienced visual improvement 8 months after surgery.

The first patient to undergo the SCOTS procedure has incrementally experienced improvements in his vision each year after repeating the procedure. He has now undergone the SCOTS procedure four times. During the 4 years he improved from sitting in a chair in his mother's house, to meeting a girl, purchasing a home, resume the practice of law (by enlarging the print on a computer), and marrying. An increasing number of patients, who have previously improved, have asked to return to repeat the surgery in the hope of achieving further visual gains.

Since the majority of our patients come to us from out of state or out of the country, much of the postoperative data are collected by a physician unrelated to us or SCOTS. In some cases, the physician has been hostile to the patient concerning their involvement in SCOTS and that makes communications difficult.

When the patient is to return home after surgery, they are given a chart detailing what testing is required at the 1-, 3-, 6-, and 12-month postoperative visits. In the past, we told the patient to ask the physician to send us the postoperative data.

In order to increase the receipt of this important information, we now instruct the patients to ask for a copy of their records at the time of their examination and send them to us. There has been an exponential increase in the number of records we now receive.

Helping patients who have never been helped before makes all the hard work extremely worthwhile.

Chapter 9
Photos

1. Arm 1

   Postoperative day #1 – The subconjunctival "hemorrhage" and inferior orbital "ecchymosis" are the bone marrow fraction or stem cell material. The actual stem cells represent a few percent of the total amount of material, which includes a myriad of growth factors. That is why I use the term "bone marrow fraction." The separation removes the red cells but the remaining material is red in color (Fig. 9.1).

Fig. 9.1 Arm 1 – postoperative day 1. (© Jeffrey N. Weiss 2020. All Rights Reserved)

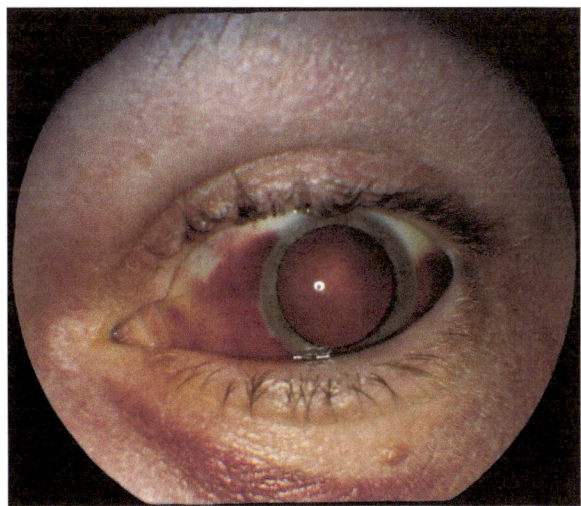

© The Author(s), under exclusive license to Springer Nature Switzerland AG 2021
J. N. Weiss, *Retinal and Optic Nerve Stem Cell Surgery*,
https://doi.org/10.1007/978-3-030-60850-7_9

2. Arm 2 – 1 day postoperatively

   (a) Intravitreal bone marrow fraction (BMF) in an eye without a posterior vitreous detachment (PVD). The stem cell material simulates a vitreous hemorrhage (Figs. 9.2 and 9.3).

   (b) Intravitreal BMF in an eye with a PVD – notice the inferior-temporal clump of material (Fig. 9.4).

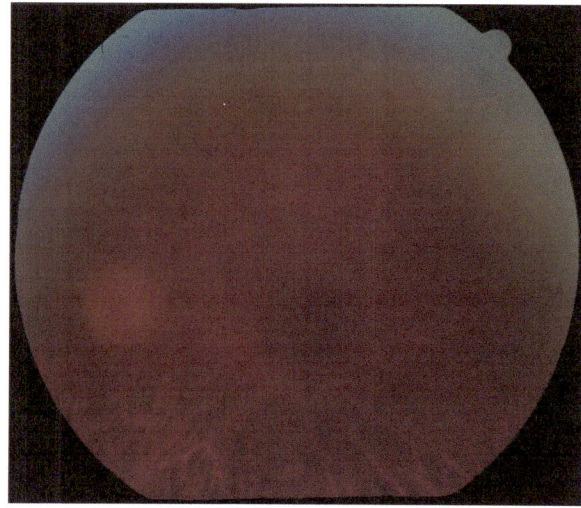

Fig. 9.2 Arm 2 – postoperative day 1. No posterior vitreous detachment. (© Jeffrey N. Weiss 2020. All Rights Reserved)

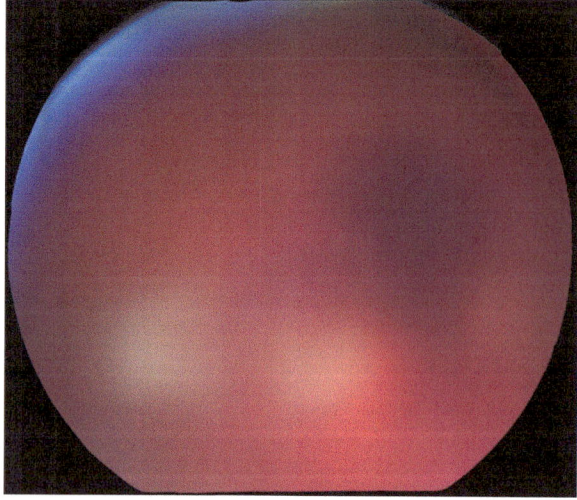

Fig. 9.3 Arm 2 – postoperative day 1. No posterior vitreous detachment. (© Jeffrey N. Weiss 2020. All Rights Reserved)

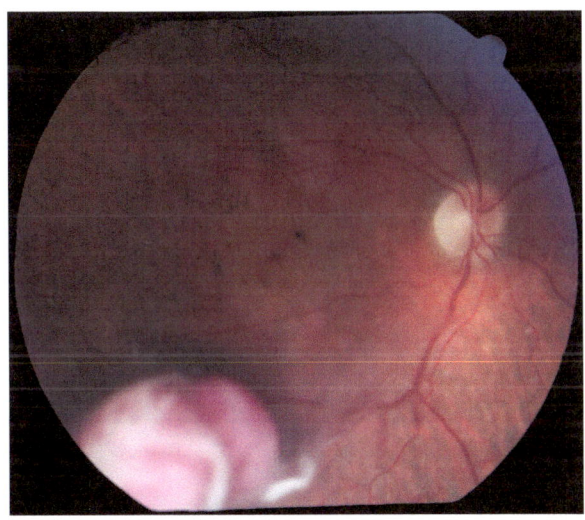

3. Arm 3
   Subretinal BMF placed in atrophic area at posterior pole

   (a) Preoperative (Figs. 9.5 and 9.6)
       In Arm 3 for AMD, the BMF is placed under the retina, and the atrophic area is filled. I use a needle I designed (manufactured by Bausch and Lomb) that makes an angled self-sealing incision in the retina. No laser photocoagulation or gas bubble is required. There have been 0 retinal detachments using this needle. However, as you will see in the subsequent photographs, the material dissipates over time. I no longer perform Arm 3 cases as the visual results are similar to those with Arm 2 or Arm 1, without the risks of performing vitrectomy surgery.
   (b) 1 day postoperative (Fig. 9.7)
   (c) 1 week postoperative (Figs. 9.8 and 9.9)
   (d) 1 month postoperative (Figs. 9.10, 9.11, 9.12, and 9.13)
   (e) 2 months postoperative (Figs. 9.14 and 9.15)
   (f) 1 day post optic nerve injection (Fig. 9.16)
   (g) Pigment clumping following Arm 3 surgery (Figs. 9.17, 9.18, and 9.19)
       There is a dissipation of the subretinal injected bone marrow fraction over several months. In some cases (above), there remains residual pigment cells. Patients with pigmentary clumps exhibit an improvement in vision, but it does not appear statistically different from those patients undergoing either an Arm 1 or Arm 2 procedure, and for this reason, I no longer perform Arm 3 surgeries.

In those cases where pigment clumps remained, there was retinal thickening as observed by ocular coherence tomography (OCT).

Fig. 9.5 Arm 3 –
preoperative. (© Jeffrey
N. Weiss 2020. All Rights
Reserved)

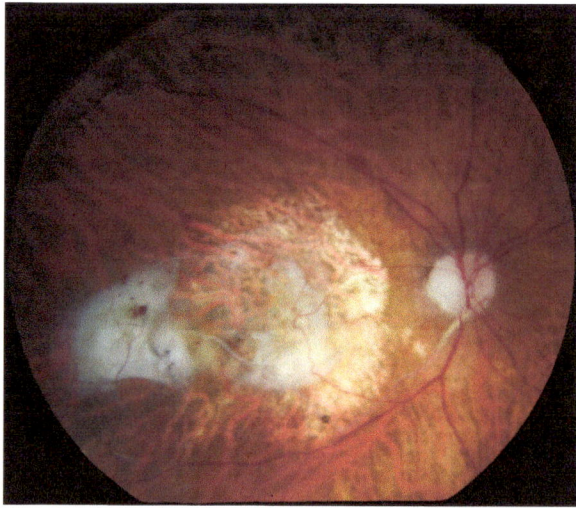

Fig. 9.6 Arm 3 –
preoperative. (© Jeffrey
N. Weiss 2020. All Rights
Reserved)

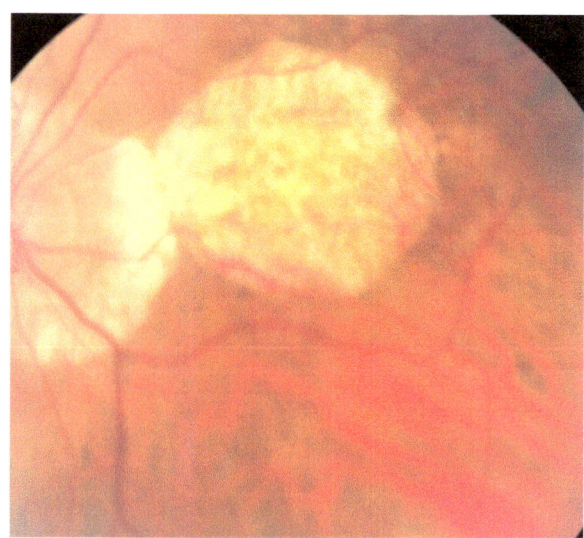

A comparison of the results from Arm 2 to Arm 1 procedures was made and no statistical difference in results was noted. For this reason, I now only perform Arm 1 surgeries.

As the results of Arm 1, Arm 2, and Arm 3 surgeries are similar, it appears that the mechanism of visual improvement is via a paracrine and not engraftment mechanism.

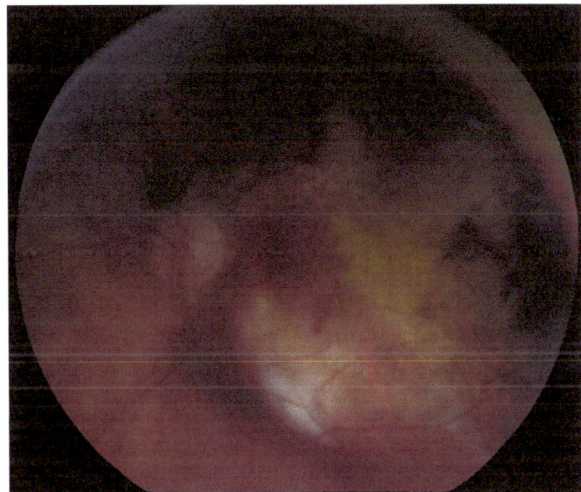

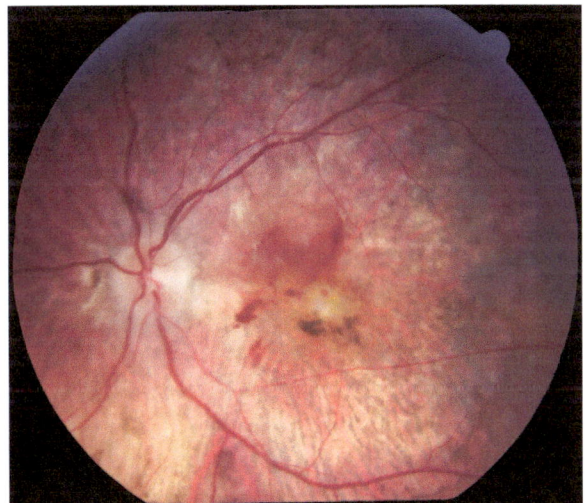

Presumably, there exist cells at the margin of those cells that are completely functioning and those that have undergone apoptosis. These cells are "idling" or in "neutral" and the SCOTS procedure potentially "re-activates" them to function. In addition, the cell activation appears to slow or preclude the progression of otherwise progressive retinal or optic nerve conditions.

Fig. 9.9 Arm 3 – 1 week
postoperative. (© Jeffrey
N. Weiss 2020. All Rights
Reserved)

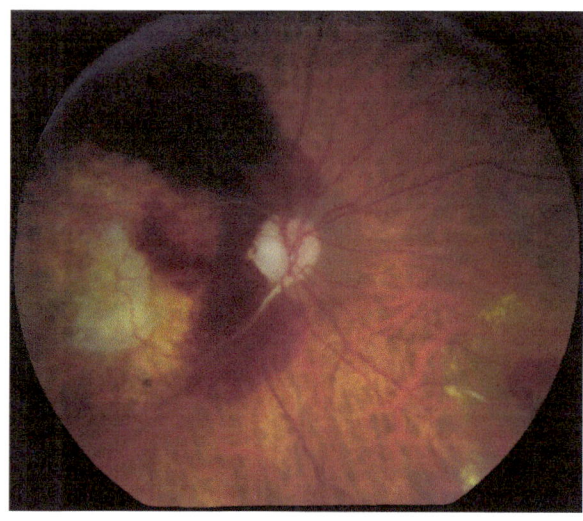

Fig. 9.10 Arm 3 –
1 month postoperative.
(© Jeffrey N. Weiss 2020.
All Rights Reserved)

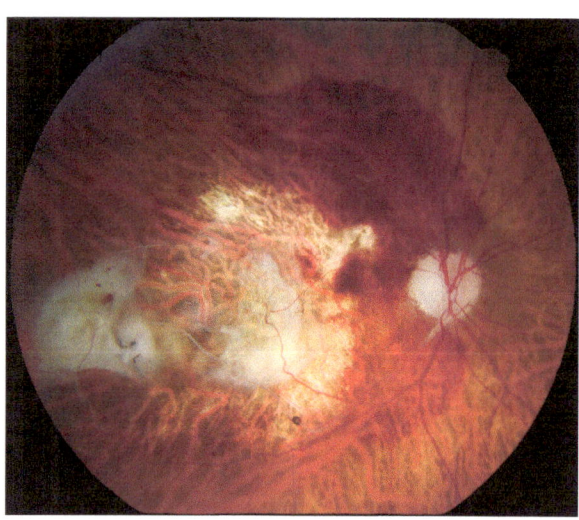

Fig. 9.11 Arm 3 –
1 month postoperative.
(© Jeffrey N. Weiss 2020.
All Rights Reserved)

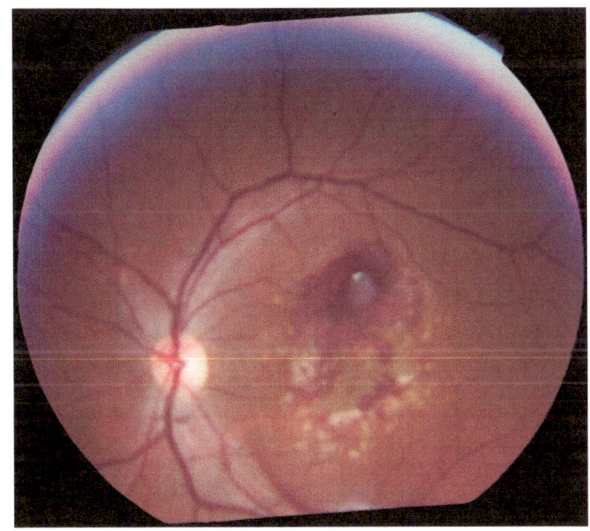

Fig. 9.12 Arm 3 –
1 month postoperative.
(© Jeffrey N. Weiss 2020.
All Rights Reserved)

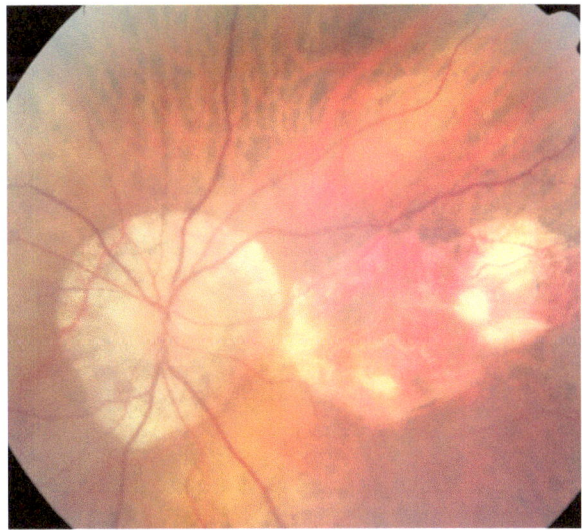

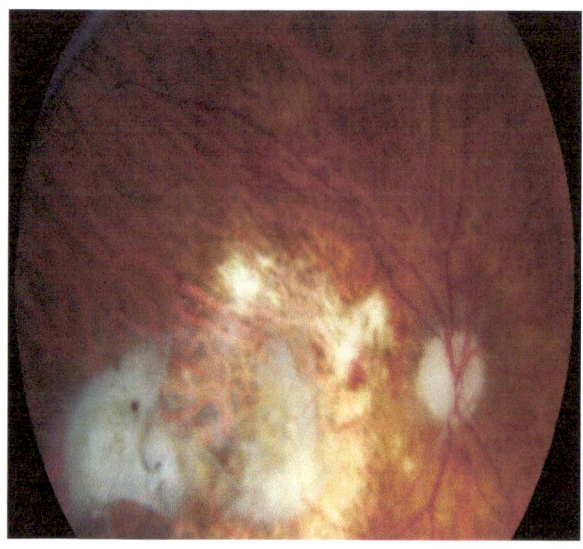

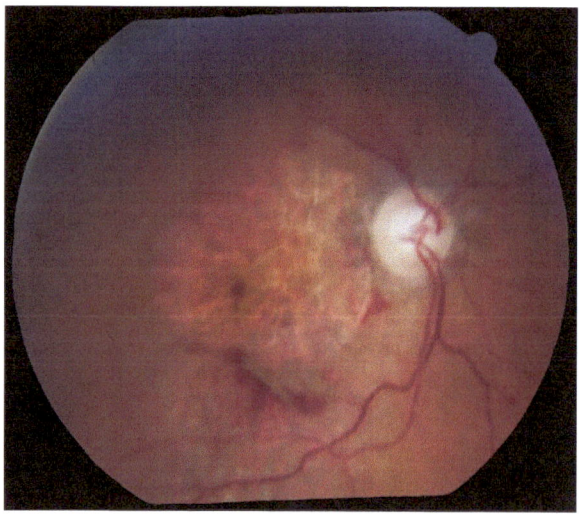

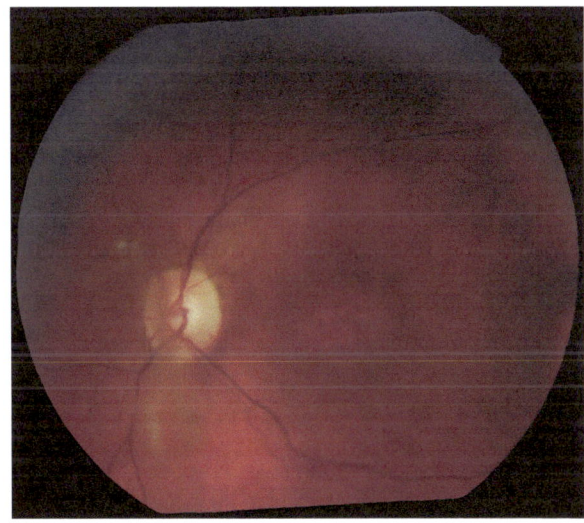

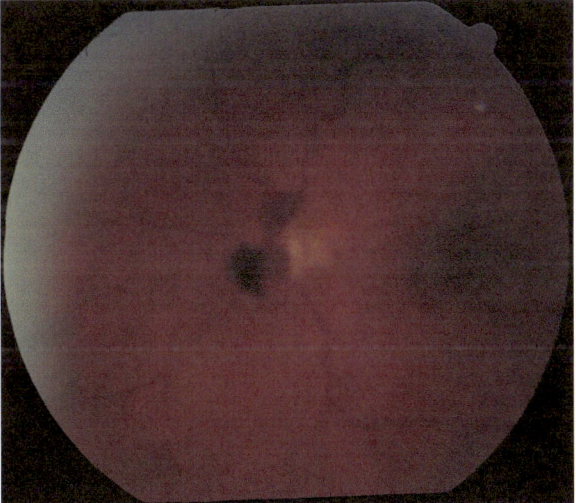

Fig. 9.17 Arm 3 –
pigment clumping.
(© Jeffrey N. Weiss 2020.
All Rights Reserved)

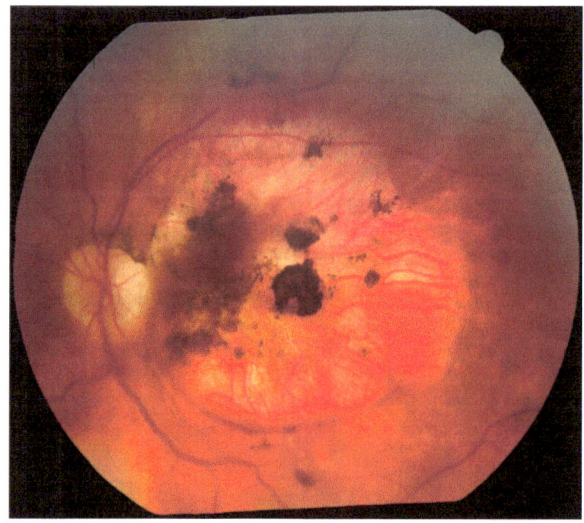

Fig. 9.18 Arm 3 –
pigment clumping.
(© Jeffrey N. Weiss 2020.
All Rights Reserved)

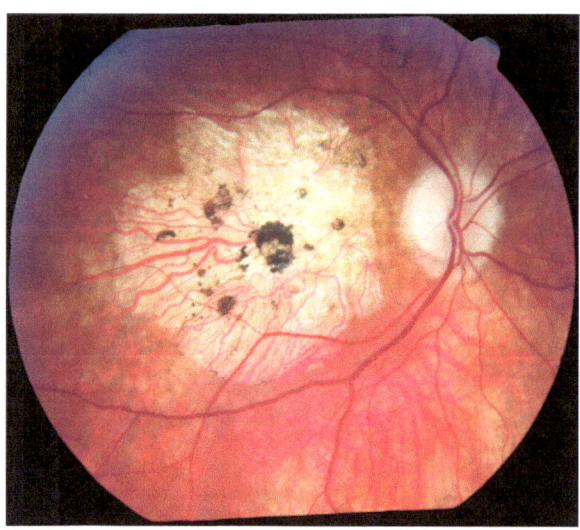

Fig. 9.19 Arm 3 – pigment clumping. (© Jeffrey N. Weiss 2020. All Rights Reserved)

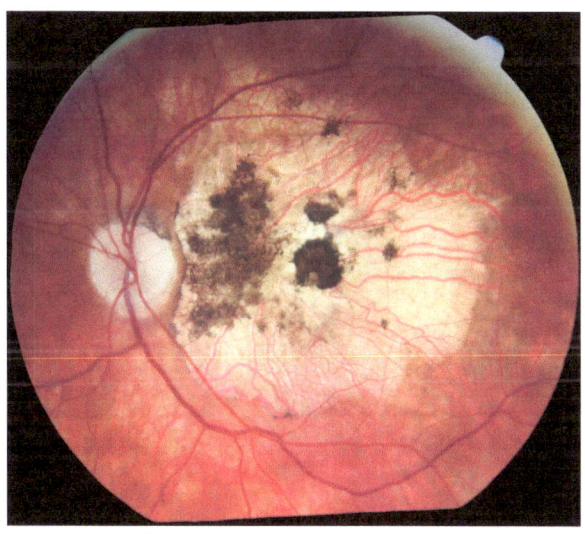

Chapter 10
Some Thoughts for the Future

Unlike pharmaceutical studies, which are tied to their methods and protocols in order to obtain FDA approval for their drug, SCOTS is a dynamic study. We can make improvements based upon experience and results. Light laser photocoagulation, as mentioned in the protocol, to aid in stem cell adherence was not found to be of benefit and is no longer performed. Likewise, subtenon steroid injections in Arm 1 or Arm 2 cases were also found not to be of benefit. An epiretinal membrane (ERM) developed in <3% of Arm 2 cases. I have not seen an ERM develop in Arm 1 cases.

There have been no complications in Arm 3 cases where I injected the optic nerve. Piercing the optic nerve was performed in radial optic neurotomy, a procedure once used in an attempt to treat central retinal vein occlusion. If the patient has sufficient vision to perform a visual field, I inject the nerve in an area without vision.

I have seen two cases (adipose derived stem cells) and have heard of several more, of patients that received VEGF inhibitors either shortly before, or after undergoing a stem cell procedure. For this reason, I will not perform the SCOTS procedure unless the patient waits at least 90 days after undergoing a VEGF inhibitor intravitreal injection. Apparently, the injection may drive the stem cells into a fibrovascular direction producing a retinal detachment.

I have investigated the use of a scaffold to aid in maintaining the subretinal stem cells in an area of atrophic retina, but at the present time, it appears that the best chance of maintaining persistence of the cells is to inject at the margin of healthy retina. Apparently, the cells are better able to adhere at the margin than at an atrophic area. But as the cells dissipate over time, and the results do not appear different between Arm 1, Arm 2, or Arm 3, I now only perform Arm 1 cases.

I have studied whether the adipose tissue found in the bone marrow aspirate (more prevalent in older patients) can affect the results but, at this time, have not found it to be the case. I also investigated multiple centrifugation cycles to improve results, but this did not appear to be of benefit.

© The Author(s), under exclusive license to Springer Nature Switzerland AG 2021   81
J. N. Weiss, *Retinal and Optic Nerve Stem Cell Surgery*,
https://doi.org/10.1007/978-3-030-60850-7_10

Quantitative Assessment

Dynamic Light Scattering

A major difficulty in retinal research is the lack of a sensitive and quantitative method to objectively determine the functional ability of the retina. Visual acuity and visual field testing are subjective methods dependent on patient response. Fundus photography, fluorescein angiography, and ocular coherence tomography (OCT) are imaging tests, which are indirectly related to functional ability and detect retinal damage relatively late in the disease process. Electrophysiologic testing is cumbersome to perform and difficult to interpret. The early detection of retinal damage at the microscopic level when it is still potentially reversible is a prerequisite for the development of advancements in therapies.

Dynamic light scattering (DLS) measures the scattered light intensity fluctuations resulting from the thermal random motion (Brownian motion) at the molecular level. The back-scattered light is recorded as a time correlation function, which relates the light intensity at time 0 to that at a chosen sample time later (1 microsecond).

Using instrumentation I developed while at M.I.T. and Harvard Medical School, DLS technology was used to predict the development of cataractogenesis in rabbits and detect diabetes mellitus in humans. The results demonstrated the utility of DLS to noninvasively quantitate subtle changes at the molecular level.

A new proof-of-concept instrument for making retinal measurements was recently developed. The original DLS device required a corneal contact lens to make the measurement. A new, upgraded, solid-state, and non-contact device has been constructed. The illumination system and the detection system were interfaced with a standard clinical fundus camera.

The scattered light was analyzed by a digital autocorrelator with an extended delay option for baseline determination. The intensity fluctuations were averaged over 2 seconds (the old device required a 5-second duration), and the cumulant analysis method used to analyze the resulting autocorrelation function and calculate the diffusion coefficient.

Preliminary pre- and postoperative measurements from patients undergoing the SCOTS procedure have detected significant quantitative improvements. A comparison of the measurements made before and 1 day after surgery demonstrated that the device was able to predict that the patient's visual acuity would improve months after the procedure. See Chap. 11 – Publication reference #8 (Fig. 10.1).

We have been using an FDA-approved Class 2 Angel device by Arthrex for stem cell and component separation. This is a centrifugal separating assembly for separating the bone marrow fraction into discrete components. The least dense particulates separate to form a top layer, and the denser components will separate and form a bottom layer. Centrifuging whole blood will result in a plasma top layer, a middle layer of white blood cells and platelets with plasma and red blood cells, known as the "buffy coat," and a bottom layer of red blood cells (Fig. 10.2).

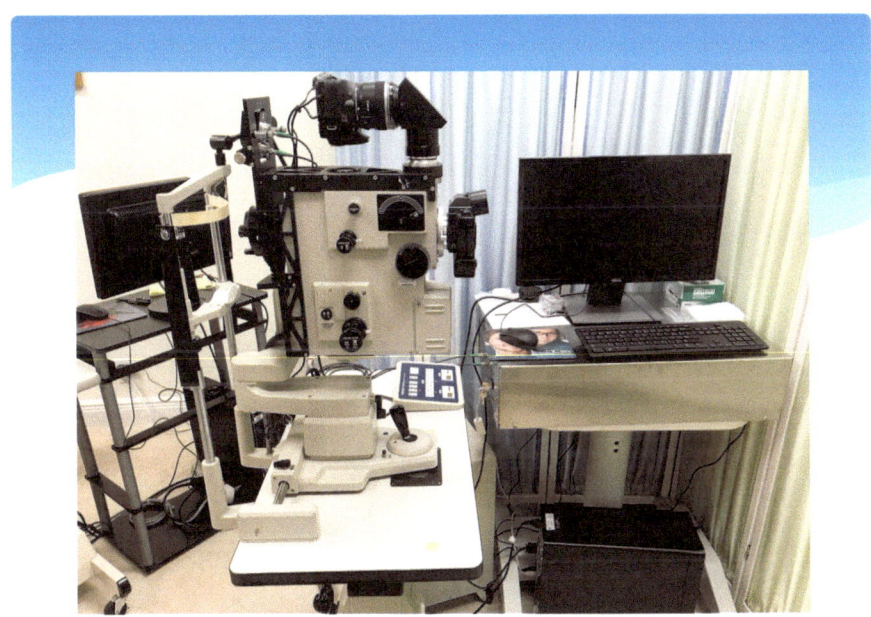

Fig. 10.1 New dynamic light scattering (DLS) device. (© Jeffrey N. Weiss 2020. All Rights Reserved)

Fig. 10.2 Bone marrow aspirate separation machine. (© Jeffrey N. Weiss 2020. All Rights Reserved)

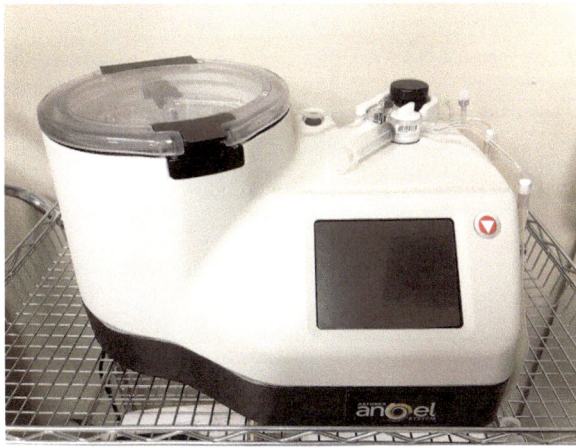

Chapter 11
Publications

Further Reading

1. Weiss JN, Levy S, Benes SC. Stem Cell Ophthalmology Treatment Study: bone marrow derived stem cells in the treatment of non-arteritic ischemic optic neuropathy (NAION). Stem Cell Investig. 2017;4:94. http://sci.amegroups.com/article/view/17421/17703.
2. Weiss JN, Levy S, Malkin A. Stem Cell Ophthalmology Treatment Study (SCOTS) for retinal and optic nerve diseases: a preliminary report. Neural Regen Res. 2015;10(6): 982–8. https://www.ncbi.nlm.nih.gov/pmc/articles/PMC4498363/.
3. Weiss JN, Levy S, Benes SC. Stem Cell Ophthalmology Treatment Study (SCOTS) for retinal and optic nerve diseases: a case report of improvement in relapsing auto-immune optic neuropathy. Neural Regen Res. 2015; 10(9): 1507–15. http://www.nrronline.org/article.asp?issn=1673-5374;year=2015;volume=10;issue=9;spage=1507;epage=1515;aulast=Weiss.
4. Weiss JN, Benes SC, Levy S. Stem Cell Ophthalmology Treatment Study (SCOTS): improvement in serpiginous choroidopathy following autologous bone marrow derived stem cell treatment. Neural Regen Res. 2016 [cited 2017 Nov 16];11:1512–6. http://www.nrronline.org/text.asp?2016/11/9/1512/191229.
5. Weiss JN, Levy S, Benes SC. Stem Cell Ophthalmology Treatment Study (SCOTS): bone marrow-derived stem cells in the treatment of Leber's hereditary optic neuropathy. Neural Regen Res. 2016;11(10):1685–94. http://www.nrronline.org/article.asp?issn=1673-5374;year=2016;volume=11;issue=10;spage=1685;epage=1694;aulast=Weiss.
6. Weiss JN, Levy S. Autologous bone-marrow derived stem cells in the treatment of "untreatable" optic nerve and retinal conditions. EC Ophthalmology. 2018;9(5):332–6. https://www.ecronicon.com/ecop/pdf/ECOP-09-00307.pdf. Summary paper.

7. Weiss JN, Levy S. Stem Cell Ophthalmology Treatment Study: bone marrow derived stem cells in the treatment of Retinitis Pigmentosa. Stem Cell Investig. 2018. http://sci.amegroups.com/article/view/19760.

8. Weiss JN, Levy S. Dynamic light scattering spectroscopy of the retina—a non-invasive quantitative technique to objectively document visual improvement following ocular stem cell treatment. Stem Cell Investig. 2019;6:8. https://www.ncbi.nlm.nih.gov/pmc/articles/PMC6509422/pdf/sci-06-2019.03.01.pdf. See Page 105.

9. Interview article with MedicalResearch.com. MedicalResearch.com - Optic nerve stroke: bone marrow stem cells provide statistically significant vision improvement   https://medicalresearch.com/stem-cells/optic-nerve-stroke-bone-marrow-stem-cells-provide-statistically-significant-vision-improvement/40837/.

10. Weiss JN, Levy S. Neurologic Stem Cell Treatment Study (NEST) using bone marrow derived stem cells for the treatment of neurological disorders and injuries: study protocol for a nonrandomized efficacy trial. Clin Trials Degener Dis. 2016 [cited 2019 Jun 18];1:176–80. http://www.clinicaltdd.com/text.asp?2016/1/4/176/196984.

11. Weiss JN, Levy S. Stem Cell Ophthalmology Treatment Study (SCOTS): autologous bone-marrow derived stem cells in the treatment of hereditary macular degeneration. EC Ophthalmol. 2019;10(7). https://www.ecronicon.com/ecop/volume10-issue7.php.

12. Weiss JN, Levy S. Stem Cell Ophthalmology Treatment Study (SCOTS): bone marrow derived stem cells in the treatment of Usher syndrome. Stem Cell Investig. 2019;6:31. http://sci.amegroups.com/article/view/29013/html.

13. Weiss JN, Levy S. Stem Cell Ophthalmology Treatment Study (SCOTS): bone marrow derived stem cells in the treatment of Dominant Optic Atrophy. Stem Cell Investig. 2019;6:41. http://sci.amegroups.com/article/view/32664.

14. Weiss JN, Levy S. Stem Cell Ophthalmology Treatment Study (SCOTS): bone marrow derived stem cells in the treatment of age-related macular degeneration. Medicines. 2020;7(4):16. https://www.mdpi.com/2305-6320/7/4/16.

Chapter 12
Frequently Asked Questions (FAQ)

1. Why do you charge patients for an "experimental" procedure?

All human endeavors, including clinical research, must be paid for. When patients think of clinical studies, they usually think of pharmaceutical companies doing research to obtain FDA approval for their drug. Pharmaceutical companies have a patent on a drug, and investments are made into research and clinical studies in hopes of obtaining FDA approval, recouping investments, and earning profits by charging patients who use the drug. SCOTS is not a patented process, there is no drug to sell. In order to provide this care and advance regenerative medicine, we must charge the patients for the procedures.

We have never had a complaint from any patient participating in these studies about our charges for the procedure. They understand the reasons for charging and that the study would not exist if no one paid.

Stem cells were discovered in 1981. SCOTS began in 2012. As of this date, there is not another study like it in the world. If SCOTS did not exist, the more than 500 patients we have treated would still not have been treated.

There is no proprietary drug at the end of the study. In fact, with the exception of the needles Dr. Weiss developed for the retinal surgery, nothing is proprietary. There is no patent protection. A pharmaceutical company cannot make a billion dollars profit, like they do with erectile dysfunction drugs. So who is to pay for it? The government?

Government funding is given to research prominent life-threatening conditions such as cancer and HIV/AIDS, and is awarded to universities and not to physicians in private practice. A private foundation? They support their own causes, have limited resources, and are guided by academics that tend to support their own, other academics. A private doctor working in his own office will not receive a grant.

Unlike a drug company study in which the treatment is free, our patients are much better informed; after all, it is their own money they are spending. Anyone has the right to spend money on anything they choose. One can purchase liquor, tobacco,

J. N. Weiss, *Retinal and Optic Nerve Stem Cell Surgery*,
https://doi.org/10.1007/978-3-030-60850-7_12

firearms, or even a house or car that they cannot safely afford without any interference. Yet, physicians who have done nothing to help these patients, who tell them to return for another visit in 6 months and charge them for the examination, only to yet again tell them that there is nothing they can do, criticize us for charging patients.

How moral is it to hold yourself out as an expert, yet be unaware of a study, listed on ClinicalTrials.gov, the NIH website, that might help the patient you are charging? And what do they offer in return? Nothing. We find it distressing that physicians who are able to see, make pronouncements about what blind patients should do, when you know that if they became blind, they would be contacting us for inclusion in our study.

2. Why are you killing babies?

The answer – we are not. This is the second most common question we hear. This work has nothing to do with embryonic or fetal stem cells. The cells we use are the patient's own stem cells – termed autologous. The bone marrow stem cells are taken from the patient during the surgical procedure.

3. Why have not you published your results in the mainstream ophthalmic journals?

We have tried. The mainstream ophthalmic journals have returned our papers without comment, or made comments we felt were inappropriate, such as personal attacks. Publishing is not free, in fact, each paper may cost us several thousand dollars to be published. That is why we are publishing in journals that are online, but are peer reviewed, and listed on the U.S. government Library of Medicine website, PubMed.gov.

Not publishing in a mainstream journal does not mean the work is not good. The reviewers are anonymous, but the authors are not. Prior studies have shown that there is bias in selecting papers for publication. Whether the authors are at a large institution, associated with the government, or at a drug company, has been found to impact the acceptance of an article. The disconnect between the research and its publication prevents the dissemination of knowledge. If publishing is the "gold standard," then the process should be transparent.

4. Why is your work considered experimental?

The definition of experimental is the use of untested ideas or techniques that are not yet established or finalized. This was true of the first cases of the many different conditions we have treated. The fact that approximately 60% of the patients have experienced visual improvement has established the idea and technique. People often criticize what they know nothing about or do not understand.

To quote Max Planck, the great German physicist,

"A new scientific truth does not triumph by convincing its opponents and making them see the light, but rather because its opponents eventually die, and a new generation grows up that is familiar with it." The history of medicine is replete with many examples of pioneers being attacked and ridiculed. The following generation of physicians, with no preconceived notions or axes to grind, accept the work.

5. Why have not you performed animal studies?

Thousands of animal studies have been performed and the data are available on PubMed, the National Library of Medicine website. Rather than reinventing the wheel, science is advanced by building on the work of others, not by repeating it. On the basis of the animal studies, various centers around the world were performing clinical studies. Dr. Weiss visited these centers and learned from them. Only then was the SCOTS protocol written and submitted to the Institutional Review Board for approval.

6. When will insurance companies pay for these procedures?

Insurance companies are profit-generating businesses. The less they pay out, the more profitable they are. Everything is experimental until there are many double-blind control clinical studies, which the insurance companies do not fund, that proves the treatment works. Since there is no funding, and it takes a generation for a new controversial medical treatment to be accepted, insurance companies will not be paying for these treatments for quite a while.

7. When will these studies end?

As long as patients are being helped, we do not expect these studies to end. And as we see improvements in other conditions, more protocols will be developed.

8. Why is the treatment so expensive?

There are many people involved in the study. The price includes payment for the anesthesiologist and his staff, Dr. Silverfarb, Dr. Levy, Dr. Weiss, the company that provides the stem cell separation equipment, the disposable equipment, the surgery center, nurses, and other personnel. We asked a university that was referring patients to SCOTS to determine what they would charge for the procedure, and they admitted that they would charge more than twice as much as we do.

9. How do patients pay for the study?

Patients typically have their own resources or have help from family or friends. Sometimes they have raised funds through donation requests through work or their religious affiliations. Not uncommonly, they have raised portions or even the entire amount through websites helping people to connect with donors such as www. gofundme.com. Patients have contacted local newspapers that have written stories about their blindness and SCOTS, which has assisted them in raising funds. Usually where there is a will, there is a way. Sadly, patient requests to prominent eye organizations, which collect millions of dollars in donations to support research involving their particular disease, have typically not resulted in any direct help for patients.

10. I heard there was a stem cell clinic in South Florida that blinded three patients.

There was a clinic in South Florida that was using adipose derived stem cells and a nurse in their office was injecting them into patient's eyes. They had a listing on clinicaltrials.gov, but that study was never performed and was withdrawn. What they were doing in their office was never IRB approved.

When I met with the FDA in 2011, they said that adipose derived stem cells were more than "minimally manipulated" and required an IND. The clinic never obtained an IND and has been closed by the FDA.

The stem cell procedures we are performing fall within FDA regulations, are FDA compliant, and do not require an IND as we are using the patient's own bone marrow, not a drug. Our studies are governed by the IRB, which is monitored by the FDA. We submit reporting to the IRB every year.

11. Are the trials on ClinicalTrials.gov vetted by the FDA?

No. The website lists trials or research studies. There are approximately 348,000 listed trials from every state and more than 200 countries. The cover page of the website clearly explains that fact.

12. Is your South Florida office the only center where you perform the procedure in the United States?

Yes. In the future, we intend to train surgeons and offer a turn-key approach including all equipment to allow physicians to perform this work. Dr. Weiss also performs surgery in Dubai, UAE.